PENGUIN ENTERPRISE

ONE WAY TO LIVE

Dr Tehemton Erach Udwadia (1934–2023) is widely considered to be the father of Indian laparoscopic surgery. As a general surgeon specializing in minimal access surgery, he popularized the procedure during a career that spanned almost seven decades and, along with his team, performed India's first laparoscopic cholecystectomy. He was the recipient of many honours, including the Padma Shri, the Padma Bhushan and the Dr B.C. Roy National Award—all of which were awarded by the President of India—and the Order of the British Empire (OBE), which was bestowed upon him by Queen Elizabeth II. He was also the president of both the Association of Surgeons of India (ASI) and the International College of Surgeons, as well as an honorary fellow of the American College of Surgeons.

In 2017, Dr Udwadia was diagnosed with a retroperitoneal leiomyosarcoma, a particularly virulent form of cancer. Over time, it became apparent to him that no more treatment options were available. Despite his grim prognosis, he elected to live life on his own terms. He continued to attend to his patients, play golf, and spend time with Khorshed, his beloved wife of sixty-four years.

He also decided to write two books about his surgical journey as a way to not just pass on the lessons he learnt from his long career, but to not dwell on his terminal illness. His first book, *More Than Just Surgery*, opened as a medical category bestseller on Amazon. This, his second book, builds on the thoughts of the first and remains a testament to his strong will. True to form, he worked until the very end, dictating the final parts of the epilogue from his hospital bed. Dr Udwadia passed away on 7 January 2023 at the hospital where he had worked for over fifty years.

He lived and worked in Mumbai.

One Way to Live

Dr Tehemton Erach Udwadia

(1934-2023)

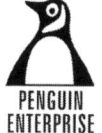

PENGUIN
ENTERPRISE

An imprint of Penguin Random House

PENGUIN ENTERPRISE

USA | Canada | UK | Ireland | Australia
New Zealand | India | South Africa | China | Singapore

Penguin Enterprise is part of the Penguin Random House group of companies
whose addresses can be found at global.penguinrandomhouse.com

Published by Penguin Random House India Pvt. Ltd
4th Floor, Capital Tower 1, MG Road,
Gurugram 122 002, Haryana, India

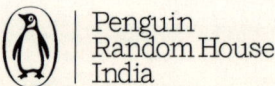

Penguin
Random House
India

First published in Penguin Enterprise by Penguin Random House India 2023

ISBN 9780143460749

Typeset in Baskerville
Printed at Replika Press Pvt. Ltd, India

www.penguin.co.in

MIX
Paper from
responsible sources
FSC® C016779

This is a legitimate digitally printed version of the book and therefore might not
have certain extra finishing on the cover.

Contents

Preface

My first book, *More Than Just Surgery*, was written with the intention of sharing what I had stumbled upon and learnt over the course of seven decades of surgery, and was a book that evolved over a protracted period of several years. *One Way to Live*, however, has been drafted with an altogether different purpose and, in some ways, is even more special than the first.

In May 2022, my wife Khorshed and I were preparing for a happy occasion in the family—our granddaughter Simone's wedding to Jamie in Manchester. The entire family, right down to grandchildren-in-law, were going to be present—an eagerly awaited family reunion! We had completed all our preparations—air tickets had been booked, saris had been packed, and *daglis* and *pagrees* were ready and waiting to be worn. But a week before our planned departure, I was admitted to the Intensive Care Unit with respiratory failure. We weren't going anywhere.

Five years ago, I had been operated upon for a nasty form of cancer, which had spread to my lungs. Of the fourteen metastases in my lungs, one was growing rapidly, which was what led to the respiratory failure, and the ICU admission that followed. The physician handling my case, perhaps anticipating that I would become a respiratory cripple, instructed me to buy an oxygen-making machine before I left the ICU—I would need supplemental oxygen whenever I left home. He was miffed when I started laughing at the thought of playing golf with a four-kilo machine strapped to my back! Later, my surgeon, a kind and gentle person, came to meet me. I asked him, 'George, surgeon to surgeon, how much time would you give me?' Without pause or hesitation, he replied, 'As surgeon to surgeon, about four to six months, give or take some.'

That evening, as I lay alone in the semi-dark ICU, with oxygen tubes in my nostrils, I made my decision. I would not lie down, a hapless captive to cancer. I would face it on my own terms. I would continue my weekly clinic at the hospital, retain my once-a-week slot in the operation theatre, and keep playing golf. For as long as I could, I would breathe without a machine. And, having gone through the struggle of writing one book, I would put myself to the ultimate acid test—I would write a second one. While I did not have the foggiest idea of what I would write about, the objective of this book would be to give me a sense of purpose, and a feeling of strength in my current situation. I was determined to take back control of my life.

But as I began the process of writing, I observed that without conscious desire or intent, this book complemented the thoughts I had expressed in the first one. *More Than Just Surgery* was about my life as a surgeon, my father's influence on me, and my despair over the surgical care of the poor, among other things. *One Way to Live* is about my personal life from childhood, my mother's influence, and my indignation at the current state of the surgical care of the aged. I have also drawn on my surgical career for a few chapters to include the setting up one of the finest surgical training centres in the world for minimal access (laparoscopic) surgery (MAS), a tribute to four hospitals (and their illustrious alums) that occupy a special place in my heart, my professional highs and lows, my thoughts on patients with cancer (being one myself), as well as a surgeon's experience of being operated upon.

Despite the fact that surgery is a team effort, with every cog in the wheel being important, the surgeon still thinks of himself or herself as the star of the show. I have learnt a great deal not only as a surgeon, but from being a surgical patient. I am convinced it would help the surgeon's growth if he or she found themselves on the other side of the table. This, and other thoughts, are detailed in this book.

With new learnings that complement the first book, *One Way to Live* had to be completed within a shorter timeframe for obvious reasons and could not have been possible without the support of my family, including my wife Khorshed, who watched in some dismay as her dining table became a drafting table once again. It could also not have been completed without a combination of push, pressure and gentle cajoling from my team, who have supported me in the writing of both my books—Titoo Ahluwalia, Gayatri Pahlajani, and Dorab Sopariwala. The team will no doubt take full responsibility for all flaws and inconsistencies herein. Surgeons, as we all know, make no mistakes.

1

The Romance

On 22 February 1949—a date I will always remember because it was exactly one month before my SSC exam—the telephone rang. I was alone at home. Mum and Dad had just left for the Thomas Cook office to finalize the itinerary of their five-and-a half-month tour of Europe and the UK; my older brother Farokh was at medical college, and my younger brother Darius was at school.

I took the call and heard a soft female voice ask, 'Who am I speaking to?'

'Tehemton Udwadia.' I replied. 'What can I do for you?'

The owner of this soft voice clearly just wanted to have a chat. We discussed which schools we were in—she, Queen Mary's and me, St Mary's—and that I was studying for my SSC exam, which was in the following month. She was yet to complete her ISC, which meant she was younger than me. I was relieved because I had thought the voice belonged to someone older. As St Mary's was a boys' school and I had no sisters, I had had no contact with girls. This was my first conversation with a girl. The conversation was pleasant and flowed freely, and when it was over, I still didn't know why she had called. I never really knew and, at the age of fourteen, I didn't really care.

Her name was Khorshed, and this would be the first of many phone conversations. And that is how our journey began. For the first month, we would speak every few days; not for too long, as I really had to study. On the last day of my SSC exams, my parents left for their foreign tour. They had arranged for Darius and I to stay with my uncle and aunt, and for Farokh and my youngest brother Firdaus, who was born in 1947, to move in with our grandparents. Once or twice a week, I would go to our home, Banoo Manor, where Khorshed would call and we would chat. There were no awkward silences; we always had enough to talk about. It was all very innocent.

Our conversations continued after my parents returned from their trip and until she left for boarding school. My parents bought me a beautiful Raleigh racer bicycle for doing well in the SSC and getting a scholarship for standing first in English in the Bombay Presidency. I joined Wilson College in June 1949 and our conversations continued till January 1951, when Khorshed was sent off to Presentation Convent, a boarding school in Kodaikanal. She looked forward to going, but was also sad we could no longer continue our conversations. She was permitted to receive letters from four people, and I was one of them. But we could not use my real name, for fear that the nuns would read the letters, so I suggested the name Tubby. I would write to her freely, but her letters to me were few and addressed to T. Udwadia at Wilson College. I was not aware that during the holidays, the college office was closed, or that the letters addressed to me would then be redirected to my home.

The first such letter redirected to my home was opened and read by Mum, and then shown to Daddy when he came home for lunch. I did not get to see the letter, but it seems it was about tennis at school and her problems with some of her school subjects. When I came home at about 7 p.m. after playing tennis at the Wilson Gymkhana, Mum seemed very angry with me, but she did not say a word. Over dinner, Daddy quietly asked me what I'd been doing that evening. Playing tennis, I replied.

With a half-smile, Daddy said, 'I am sure all your games were love games.'

Mum exploded. 'Erach, don't try to make a joke out of your son's disgraceful behaviour,' she said to Daddy. 'No wonder after such good results in the SSC, he did so poorly next year in his college exams. He had no mind for his studies.' Her long tirade continued even after the plates had been cleared. Farokh and Darius walked away, but I couldn't. I knew that although Daddy didn't say anything, they were both very upset with me. In conservative Parsee families in the 1950s, the concept of a sixteen-year-old boy having a girlfriend was not acceptable. Mum took Khorshed's home number from me and telephoned her mother. That was the end of all contact between Khorshed and me for more than a year.

Meanwhile, I got into GS Medical College in the same year, 1951. Khorshed returned from boarding school at the end of 1953 after her Senior Cambridge exam, but Mum took no chances. She shifted our telephone from the sitting room to her bedroom and would lock the room when she went out. But I found the spare key in a desk in her bedroom, took it before she left, and replaced it after she got back. Khorshed's and my conversations continued willy-nilly.

Around March 1954, we began wondering if we should meet. That required courage because if someone saw us and word got back to my mother, the result would be catastrophic. In addition, I was worried that if Khorshed was a short, fat, cross-eyed girl with thick glasses and pimples, I would not be able to extricate myself from the situation without hurting her feelings. Later, she told me she had similar concerns about me!

Putting aside all our worries, we decided to meet on 8 April. I was nineteen and she was eighteen. It had to be at a place where no one could recognize us. Khorshed said that Kemp and Company, a pharmacy at Kemps Corner, would be empty in the afternoon. We decided to meet there at 2.45 p.m. and then go for a movie to the New Empire cinema.

I was in charge of the logistics. My classmate from GS Medical College, Robin d'Andrade, lived close to New Empire and I tasked him with the responsibility of purchasing two one-rupee-four-anna tickets for the 3.30 p.m. show, and to make sure that the seats were as inconspicuous as possible. It was a rule amongst our friends that all transactions between us were on a cash-on-delivery basis. So when he handed me the tickets on the fifth, I had to fork out two rupees and eight annas to him, then and there. That burned a big hole in my ten-rupee budget—it was two months' pocket money for me. I hid the two tickets between the pages of the surgery textbook *Rose and Carless.**

Our 2.45 p.m. meeting would give me enough time to be present for the ward clinics till 1 p.m. and still reach New Empire by 3.30 p.m. I wore my best shirt, an Arrow that my mother had bought in Ceylon during our holiday there the previous year, along with white trousers and old but well-polished shoes.

Immediately after my morning ward round, I went to my friend Eddie D'Souza's room in the GS Medical College hostel—that was our group's clubhouse—to iron my shirt. I then took the train from Elphinstone Road to Grant Road and walked towards Kemps Corner. I was fifteen minutes early and did not know what to do, so I crossed the road and went into an Irani restaurant called Mazda, and sat at a table. The waiter asked for my order. I didn't want to spend any money, so I told the waiter I was waiting for a friend and would place the order after he came.

When it was nearly 2.45 p.m., I quietly slipped out of the restaurant. As I entered Kemp and Company, I first saw a short salesman with a white shirt and a black tie and then, at the opposite counter, a girl. I was so flabbergasted that I felt my legs wobble and had to clutch the counter for support. I had never imagined that such a beautiful girl could exist! She was tall, had a sweet smile, and had lovely brown hair that hung below her shoulders. The corners of her lips were twitching slightly; I realized she was nervous, and I wanted to

---

* William Rose, *Rose and Carless's Manual of Surgery* (Bailliere: Tindall and Company, 1944).

reassure her. She was wearing a yellow dress made out of a dimpled fabric, a broad black leather belt with a shiny buckle that accentuated her slim waist, and black shoes that also had shiny buckles. Hanging from one wrist was a black purse in the shape of a box with a metal clasp. Her outfit was perfectly matched. There was something special about her, and I knew then that she was the one I wanted to spend the rest of my life with.

She walked up to me and in a soft, melodious voice said, 'I am Khorshed, and it is such a pleasure to meet you.'

Meanwhile, the salesman was obviously annoyed that we were using his pharmacy as a rendezvous spot. 'Why are you here? What have you come for? What do you want to buy?' he asked me loudly. That brought me back to earth. 'I want a child's toothbrush,' I said, thinking that would be the cheapest item in the shop. The salesman put a small green toothbrush on the counter and said, 'One rupee'.

I was sure he had increased the price out of spite, but I had no choice. With a heavy heart, I parted with the rupee. I now had six rupees and eight annas for the rest of the evening. Since the unsporting salesman with no feeling for romance was almost certainly going to throw us out of the shop, we left. And outside, my legs started wobbling again. In the sunlight, I saw that Khorshed had brown eyes and her hair had a touch of brown and gold!

We walked to the B-route bus stop, not knowing when the next bus would come. This was the first time Khorshed would be travelling by bus and she was excited. When the double-decker arrived, we sat on the lower deck. The conductor turned the handle of his machine and two tickets of two annas each rolled out. We got down at the stop closest to New Empire.

I gave the doorman our two tickets and I started walking down the aisle. 'Come back, sir', the doorman said, pointing to the only two seats in the last row, next to the exit. My heart sank. Those were the two most conspicuous seats in the theatre! Anyone going out during the interval would be able to see who was sitting there. I cursed Robin for his weird sense of selection and sat on the aisle seat, praying that none of my mother's friends were around.

The movie that afternoon was *Decameron Nights*, which was about the nightly exploits of some semi-demented Don Juan. Before it came on, there were the usual Indian news, Movietone news, and trailers of forthcoming movies. At the interval, we were faced with Hobson's choice. Should we sit where we were—on the only two seats in the last row right next to the exit—and risk being spotted, or go out into the lobby and risk being spotted there?

Khorshed decided it was better to remain in place and talk. I said I had a present for her and gave her the toothbrush I'd purchased! Incidentally, since then, I've only used green toothbrushes. She said she also had a present for me and took out two sets of plastic shirt buttons from her purse. At the time, such buttons were often used in place of stitched buttons. My gift was costlier than hers.

The seats in the row in front of us were empty and we chatted gaily in whispers throughout the movie, just as we'd always done over the telephone. Whenever we looked up to see what was happening in the movie, we saw scenes of men jumping off balconies onto horses standing below and galloping away, or sword fights, or angry husbands chasing the hero or villain. The second the movie was over, we bolted away from the crowd.

After a while, we found ourselves near the Eros theatre. Whenever I played cricket matches at the Oval Maidan and lunch was included, we would go to the restaurant on the first floor of the Eros building. Their prices were reasonable. I calculated quickly: I had six rupees and four annas left. That was enough for two teas and a plate of sandwiches. But what if she wanted a milkshake or a chocolate cake?

Anyway, the die had been cast. I took the risk and we entered the near-empty restaurant. When I gave the order, Khorshed said she didn't drink tea. Once again, my heart sank. Did she want some expensive drink? To my immense relief, she said she wasn't thirsty or hungry. She looked even more beautiful to me when she said that! I had the tea and three sandwiches, and I even managed to persuade her to have one. I now had two rupees left.

We walked out of Eros, crossed Churchgate Station and once on Queen's Road, took the broad, pleasant walkway alongside the railway track. Alas, over the years, this walkway kept shrinking as more and more tracks were laid to accommodate the ever-increasing local train traffic. It was past 7 p.m. by then and we continued walking, talking and laughing until we reached Opera House.

I had never travelled by taxi, so I knew practically nothing about the fares. Still, I was sure that cabbing it from Opera House to Kemps Corner would be less than two rupees. Pretending that I'd just realized it was late, I told Khorshed, 'I am so sorry! I made you walk all this way not realizing how late it is. Let's get a taxi and I will drop you home.'

When the taxi stopped outside her home in Nazir House, just a few buildings beyond Kemps Corner, she opened the door, turned, lightly touched me on my arm, and thanked me for a wonderful evening. After getting out and taking a few steps, she turned, waved to me and then walked in.

Just in case she was watching, I asked the driver to start and take a U-turn. That would suggest that I was taking the taxi home. But as soon as Khorshed was out of sight, I asked the cabbie to stop and got out. The fare was 10 annas. I had more than a rupee left!

I pretty much ran all the way home—a distance of about a mile. I knew my mother would be annoyed and interrogate me as to why I was returning so late from a 3.30 p.m. movie. But I was lucky. She had been irritated but had then phoned Robin's house and was told by his mother that Robin had taken two rupees and eight annas from her a few days earlier for two movie tickets, and so she assumed that Robin and I had gone together. That had calmed and reassured her, and the wonderful day ended on a very pleasant note.

After dinner, as I lay in bed and relived the day I'd had, I realized that despite almost six hours together, the only physical contact between Khorshed and me had been her light touch on my arm as she had got out of the taxi. Yes, romance moved gently and slowly in the 1950s. That perhaps strengthened it and made it last.

After that first time together, we would meet every ten to fifteen days. We would rendezvous outside Kemp and

Company and walk up the slope to Hanging Gardens. At 2.30 in the afternoon, the gardens would be deserted and hot. We would sit in the shade of a tree on the wooden benches. Once, we went to the Kamala Nehru Park across the road and saw the gorgeous views of Chowpatty, Colaba and the islands beyond the Gateway of India. But the park had been full of schoolchildren, so we didn't go there again.

From Hanging Gardens, we would walk down to Nepean Sea Road, and I would show her 'Citadel', the large five-to-six-storey building constructed by Minoo uncle, my mother's brother. We also found a small lane with bungalows. One had a large wooden gate with a board saying 'Bon Espoir'. Thanks to my SSC French, I knew that 'Bon Espoir' meant 'Good Hope'. We decided to adopt 'Bon Espoir' as our motto.

I felt these secret meetings could not be sustained, so I decided to tell my mother about us. Occasionally, Mum and I would go to Hanging Gardens too. On one such trip, whilst we were enjoying the view, I summoned all my courage and told her that I had met the girl I used to talk to on the phone when I was in Wilson College. Mum didn't show any emotion. She just said, 'Let's go home,' and we drove back in complete silence.

After dinner, she, Dad and I sat in their bedroom and in a soft voice, she told me that I must think of my future as a doctor, or perhaps as a surgeon. She pointed out that in my first-year exam at Wilson College, I'd got a third class, but once she'd cut off my contact with Khorshed, I did very well in my inter exams, but then failed in my first year MBBS exams when I resumed talking to her. She explained that studying medicine was a full-time activity and that Khorshed's family and ours were very different. We were respectable professionals, whereas Khorshed's father imported foreign cars, owned racehorses and had made a fortune during the last war, trucking goods and soldiers for the British Army. If Khorshed and I married, her family would pull me out of medical college and make me sell cars and horses. Our family dream of my becoming a doctor and following in my father's footsteps would be shattered. Therefore, she said, she would explain to Khorshed's mother that our friendship had to end immediately.

I was heartbroken and wished I had not opened my big stupid mouth at Hanging Gardens. Starting at the end of June 1954, there was a total embargo on our meeting or talking. Then in early October, the phone rang, and it was Khorshed, saying that she would be attending a sports event I was participating in. 'I will be at the University Athletics final day,' she said. Before my mother could see I was on the phone, I immediately disconnected.

The event was always held at the Cooperage grounds. Students from every college would be there. For the first time in recent memory, the GS Medical College was in the finals of the 4x100m relay. Our team comprised Clive Martin, Behrooz (Broozy) Irani, another Irani boy whose name I cannot remember now but whose father owned one of the largest Irani restaurants near the Metro Cinema, and myself. We had cleared three qualifying rounds to enter the finals. Clive and I were the fastest ones on our team, so I took the first run, the two Irani boys went next, and Clive ran the last leg. We stood fourth.

After removing my shorts and spikes and changing into regular clothes, I started looking for Khorshed. Someone tapped my shoulder. It was her. She had driven in a smart new Austin car. We drove around for a while and then entered a vast open area in the military cantonment with a 'No Entry' sign outside. We hugged and kissed but soon got scared and decided to leave. As we were driving out, we saw other cars with couples driving in!

After that reunion in late 1954, we started meeting every three or four weeks. We couldn't meet more frequently because my final MBBS exams were coming up and I had to clear seven subjects in one go. I was sure that by now, Mum and Dad were probably aware that Khorshed and I were still meeting, but they saw me studying very hard, and perhaps did not want to rock the boat.

While I was studying in medical college, Khorshed joined St Xavier's College in 1953 but quit after eight months. She preferred taking the full-time courses at the Young Women's Christian Association (YWCA) in shorthand, typing and accounts, which she felt would be of more use to her than studying Shakespeare's *The Merry Wives of Windsor* for an entire year (the course entailed studying one play a year). After these classes, she took cooking lessons from Villie Mehta and continued her piano lessons, but right from her time at Presentation Convent, Khorshed's passion had been tennis. Every weekday, for almost two hours, she would take tennis lessons at the Western India Automobile Association (WIAA) Club (now known as the Malabar Hill Club) from Mr Solanki, the club's head coach, and reached a level of proficiency where she could compete at local, state, and national levels.

I did well in my final year of MBBS. This guaranteed that I would be able to get a seat for the Master's in Surgery course at the King Edward Memorial (KEM) Hospital and become a surgeon. That gave me the leverage to ask my parents for permission to get engaged to Khorshed. After Dad persuaded Mum that, contrary to her expectations, Khorshed had been a stabilizing and motivating force for me, Mum agreed. We were engaged on 12 February 1957, which was the second month of my very first Resident's post at Wadia Children's Hospital.

Now we could meet freely, but I was on call at the hospital six days a week. Subhash Dalal, my registrar, very kindly took two of those calls, thus enabling Khorshed and I to meet at least twice a week. Khorshed's parents had a fabulous sprawling beach house in Juhu, right in front of the beach. When we had the car, we'd drive to Juhu, passing by paddy fields with small houses, and another pretty cottage called 'The Jet' along the way. The only shop on our route was Solomon's Mines, a well-known antiques shop.

Over time, as I continued my surgical residency, Khorshed's parents felt that since we had known each other for nine years, we should get married at the earliest. But my mother was totally against the idea—she said that because I was younger than Farokh, I couldn't marry before him. Moreover, she was convinced that if I married Khorshed, I would fall completely under the influence of Khorshed's parents and would never complete my MS degree.

It was then that Khorshed's father, Ratoo, hit on an ingenious plan. He and Khorshed's mother, Jaloo, came to our home unannounced one afternoon. Mum was alone. Over tea, Ratoo asked Mum in a hushed voice if she had noticed that I had packed a suitcase. My mother was puzzled. Ratoo then told her that I had got a very good job as a tea plantation doctor in the Nilgiris, and that he felt that Khorshed and I were secretly planning to elope. My mother's face grew ashen—to a respectable Parsee family in the 1950s, the stigma of elopement would always haunt them. However, Ratoo continued, if my mother agreed to the marriage, he would make sure I'd continue my studies and become a surgeon.

Mum had been pushed into a corner from which there was no escape. It was decided that our wedding would take place in early January 1959.

2

The Udwadia Saga

It took Khorshed and me five years—from 1949 to 1954—to meet for the first time, and another five years to get married. When we started our courtship in February 1949, I was fourteen and she was thirteen. By the time our wedding was fixed for 5 January 1959, I was twenty-four and she was twenty-three. By then, we had known each other for ten long, happy, intermittently rocky, unforgettable years.

At that time, Allbless Baug was a sought-after wedding venue for Parsees in Bombay,* and one had to draw lots to reserve it. My mother, Khorshed's mother and our aunts went multiple times to draw lots, all without success. So we opted for the Seth Jeejeebhoy Dadabhoy Agiary ground as our wedding venue. Now a beautiful location by the sea in Colaba, it was seldom used at the time and was barren and undeveloped. Those were the days of strict prohibition but to Khorshed's father, no Parsee celebration was complete without free-flowing alcohol. This shocked and scared the law-abiding Udwadia family, but Ratoo would not budge.

---

* *Interchangeably used with Mumbai throughout this book.*

We got married on a cold, windy day and while the wedding was being solemnized by the priests, I could feel Khorshed shivering against my shoulder as we sat next to each other during the ceremony. I think it was a happy wedding, with alcohol adding to the boisterousness. As I was the first from my batch to get married, a large number of guests were my college friends. My wedding pagree was passed around like a package, had several falls, and was eventually deformed and dented. Uma Sami, a special college friend, sang our song 'Softly, Softly' on the microphone. At one point, Broozy (from our relay team) asked us where the photographer was. I asked Khorshed, she asked her mother, who asked her father. Photographer? No one had thought of a photographer! Broozy, who lived nearby, rushed home, fetched his box camera, got Khorshed and me to stand on the stage and took one picture. To date, it is the *only* picture we have of our wedding.

As a newly married couple, we had a relatively luxurious start to life. We moved into Khorshed's parents' old apartment in Nazir House. Her parents used her recently matured insurance policy to buy us a small Standard car. My salary as an Indian Council of Medical Research (ICMR) fellow at the time, was 400 rupees a month and petrol was four rupees a gallon (not litre). The day before the wedding, I took my most valuable possessions with me to Nazir House—my small steel cupboard for my clothes, a Retina camera my parents had bought for me on their Europe trip in 1949, a small Remington typewriter, a table lamp Farokh and I shared on our common study table, a small leatherbound Parsee prayer book gifted to me on the occasion of my Navjote in

April 1941 by Perry & Company Chemists (which supplied Daddy's medicines) with my name embossed in gold, and a warm, loving and long letter written to me by Darius on the day before the wedding. The last two remain in my dressing-table drawer till today.

Khorshed put her courses in shorthand, typing and accounts management to good use. Every item bought (from mutton at four rupees a pound to cinema tickets at one rupees and four annas per ticket) was meticulously recorded, and at the end of each month, she ensured we had saved money from my salary. She took shorthand dictation of my notes and typed them out on the Remington. When the time came, Khorshed also typed the dissertations for my Fellowship of College of Physicians and Surgeons (FCPS) and MS theses. These were eventually bound into books by Mr Godia, the GS Medical College typist, who must have done the same for hundreds of students over the course of his thirty-year career. It was around this time that we also got a dog called Happy.

The next addition to our family was our firstborn Rushad, who was born on 19 February 1960, a few days before I took up my registrar post at the KEM Hospital with Dr P.K. Sen. In those days, mothers were required to stay in the hospital for over two weeks after delivery. With Khorshed in the hospital and me stuck with my books, studying for the MS examination until late at night, our dog Happy was distinctly unhappy. One night, at about 3 a.m., after I finished studying, I saw him lying at my feet, listless. Feeling sorry for him, I picked him up and drove the two-minute distance to the Parsee General Hospital where Khorshed was.

She had a large room in the Obstetrics (OB) ward along the front veranda. There was no air conditioning back then, and the doors were wide open, the curtains gently billowing in the breeze. Khorshed was in bed and Rushad was in a cot next to the ayah, who was asleep. I held Happy tightly in my arms. He wriggled with joy when he saw Khorshed but made no sound. I tiptoed to the cot and lifted the mosquito net to let Happy see Rushad. Wagging his tail furiously, he took a long, quiet look. I was about to replace the mosquito net, when the ayah awoke and, thinking I was stealing Rushad, started screaming hysterically, '*Chor! Chor! Bachche ko chori karta hai! Pakro!*' (Thief! Thief! Catch him, he's stealing the baby!) Every light in every room in the corridor came on. In the dim light, the ayah thought the dog in my arms was Rushad. Mothers, nurses, ayahs and ward boys suddenly besieged me. Happy started barking furiously—it was a scene from a lunatic asylum. When I came to visit Khorshed the next evening, this time without Happy, there was a freshly painted notice by the hospital steps: 'Dogs not allowed'.

I became a first-time father in February, joined Professor Sen's team as his registrar in March, passed the FCPS exam in April, and was keen to do my MS in May. Professor Sen tried to dissuade me, saying I was trying to take on too much at one time. Of course, I didn't listen, and appeared for and failed the MS exam. Surprisingly, however, I was not greatly traumatized by the failure. With Khorshed's cheerful attitude and Rushad to boost my morale, I cleared the MS exam the next time. The following May, Dinaz was born. With two children under the age of two, Khorshed had her hands full.

Time cannot and does not stand still—the next phase involved moving first to Ireland, and then to the UK, for the FRCS exam and further training. Till we were settled in Ireland, we left the children in the care of Khorshed's parents, and our dog Happy with my parents. A couple of nights before we were due to leave for Ireland, Dr Khurshed Sahiar, my co-resident pathologist at the KEM Hospital dropped by with a blank form in his hand and requested me to sign it. It was a form for the membership of the Willingdon Club. I burst into laughter— living hand to mouth, how could I join the elite Willingdon Club? He explained that my turn to become a member would come only after a few years, well after I returned to India from Ireland. If I filled the form now, I was not required to pay anything immediately and the fees would be low too. I was called for the membership interview in 1965, two years after my return from England. The fee was a staggering 30,000 rupees, but I was allowed to pay in three yearly instalments of 10,000 rupees each. Membership to the Willingdon opened up the joys of golf to me. For over fifty-five years, I have walked on the grass, surrounded by trees, birdsong and flowers, playing with friends who have grown old with me. Golf teaches one everything there is to know about life—about its ups and downs, about how to recover from failure, and about fair play. It is a great leveller, inviting you to play not against your opponent, but against the golf course and yourself. I never fail to bless Dr Sahiar, who made access to this world possible for me.

But for now, Ireland beckoned. Cheaper to live in and an easier place to pass the Primary FRCS from, Dublin became our first stop. We grew to love Ireland and the Irish, and subsequently enjoyed several motoring holidays around the country. Our landlady was a Mrs Kay Mills, a warm, friendly and generous lady. Two other students of the Primary FRCS were in the next room: Dr Parlevil from Colombo and Dr Nambiar from Madras. It was a great help to have them there. After studying late into the night, we would all go to the kitchen, make tea, have biscuits and discuss various topics. The midnight feast was not part of our agreement, but Mrs Mills pretended to take no notice.

One night, at about 1 a.m., we heard banging on our bedroom door. It was Parlevil and Nambiar, who were both in a state of panic. Parlevil had been washing his shirt in their shared basin, which had suddenly come off the wall. Pipes and water were splattered all over the floor. What were we to do? We left the matter to Khorshed. While we were at college, she told Mrs Mills about the debacle. Mrs Mills took it in her stride and arranged for two engineers—her regular paying guests from Belfast, who were already coming over to stay—to install a new basin, fix the pipes, the works. She did not charge for the basin, and the engineers did not charge for their work. That was Ireland back then.

But we soon found a way to reciprocate her generosity. Mrs Mills used to dye her hair a lovely dark brown and after one such occasion, she knocked on our door early on the following morning. She was wheezing, struggling to breathe, her face and neck swollen, puffy and red. She had had an allergic reaction to the dye. The cost of medical care in Ireland was very high in those days but luckily for Mrs Mills, Parlevil was asthmatic and had brought steroids with him. I had antihistamines. Between us, we looked after her for three to four days, until she was well. Toast, butter and jam were added to our midnight snacks.

With the Primary FRCS cleared in Dublin, we sent for the kids and moved to Edinburgh to prepare for the Final FRCS. Our move coincided with the Edinburgh Festival, so finding affordable accommodation was nearly impossible. We finally found a small apartment in the Sciennes Road area, and its only advantage was that it had a basin, a toilet and a bathtub— the only apartment in the vicinity with all these facilities; our neighbours had to use a large block of communal washrooms. We were amazed at how primitive Edinburgh was in 1962. The cold winds would sweep in from under the door of our ground-floor apartment, lift the linoleum off the floor and ensured that we shivered. It also didn't help that the apartment came with an inexplicable clothesline full of ladies' bras and underwear hung from wall to wall.

It took us two days to clean up the mess, nail down the linoleum firmly to the floor, and board up the front door to keep the wind out. Edinburgh may or may not have contributed to making me a surgeon, but it ensured I got a crash course in becoming a handyman. There were only two beds, and a cot for one-year-old Dinaz was a must, so I bought a cot and mattress for £2.50 from a hardware store, but had to assemble the cot myself. Transporting the cot and mattress was another £2.50, which was more than our daily expenditure at the time, and it was then I put my foot down. If I could be a handyman, I could also be a coolie. I walked the one and a half miles back to our apartment carrying the cot and mattress on my head through the streets of Edinburgh—money saved, new skill acquired.

Once we settled in, I would study until 2-3 a.m. Very often in the middle of the night, there would be a knock on the door. Khorshed's father Ratoo was not in the best of health and the only mode of communication available at the time was telegram. I would rush to the door in the bitter cold, wearing the huge coat my father had bought to keep himself warm on his Europe holiday in 1949, to find a different man on the pavement each time. 'Is Susan in?', he would ask. The next time, another enquiry, 'Is Janet free?' This was how we learnt that our apartment, located conveniently at street-level, had formerly been a brothel.

With no job and our bank balance plunging to new depths, I wrote to Khorshed's parents requesting them to send air tickets for her and the children to fly back home. But by an act of God and the intervention (unknown to me at the time) of my Bombay chief at the KEM Hospital, Professor P.K. Sen, I secured a registrar's job in a teaching hospital in Liverpool, a small miracle for an Indian surgeon who had yet not completed his FRCS! While I had yet to complete my FRCS in Edinburgh, I could study from Liverpool.

Life in Liverpool was joyfully different. We had a large apartment in a good, quiet locality, Fairfield Crescent, with an old, refined landlady. Our bedroom was on the second floor, the kitchen and sitting room on the third floor, and the washroom on the first. The only heating was by coal fire in the fireplace in the bedroom, and an electric heater in the compact kitchen. While I would enthusiastically bring two buckets of coal from the garage to the bedroom, the real job of starting the fire was Khorshed's. She would struggle for an hour to get the fire started, using newspapers, wood, coal and even kerosene, her hands and face smeared with soot by the time she was done. It was a miracle that she did not burn the house down. But once she learnt to light the fire, we began to appreciate the joy of a fireplace in a cold, wet country. Khorshed made friends with the grocer, the butcher, the baker and with my steady income, we felt better about life. She would trot off to the laundrette in her high heels with the two children in a double pram, or to nearby Sefton Park. I would study late into the night in the small kitchen, kept warm by the electric heater. Things were beginning to turn around.

As I was on call at the hospital five days a week, owning a car was a necessity to attend to emergencies. As soon as I started the job, I got a third- or fourth-hand Ford for £105. Mrs Robinson, our landlady, was aloof and we felt she was lonely. The evening I got the car, I told my wife and children that we would go for a drive. Khorshed suggested we take Mrs Robinson along on our first drive. Mrs Robinson came up to the car in a fur coat, a fur cap and fur gloves. We thought she was dressed to meet the Queen, but she had to settle for the Udwadias. We had a refreshing hour-long drive, past the huge Kraft factory and into the outskirts of Liverpool. Khorshed's suggestion to include Mrs Robinson in our little life event ensured that she became a part of our family.

The winter of 1962 was the most severe the UK had seen in sixty years. From October, instead of two buckets of coal, I had to carry three from the garage. A small oil lamp was put under the engine of my old Ford to make sure the engine was 'awake' in the morning. The water heater was kept on for most of the night to make sure the water pipes did not freeze and burst. Mrs Robinson spent Christmas and New Year every year with her daughter in Manchester, and was planning to leave on 17 December, which created a problem for us. The Edinburgh FRCS was starting on 3 January 1963, and I could not possibly leave Khorshed and the children alone in a freezing house. So I booked a hotel for them while I was away for the exam. When Mrs Robinson heard of this, she cancelled her plans and decided to stay back in Liverpool with Khorshed and the children, and this is something we will never forget. In the end, none of us felt the cold for the simple reason that I passed the Edinburgh FRCS and later the English FRCS in London in May!

My next position as a registrar at the Royal Liverpool Hospital was more than just educative. It gave me an overview of how surgery was practised in western countries and added sophistication to my approach. But by June, I was raring to return to Bombay. We sent the children back with Khorshed's parents who had come to the UK to visit us. We were now ready for our six-week holiday in Europe, just the two of us. We had saved £350 and decided to splurge—or as much as a young couple could afford to splurge in Europe. Over the ensuing six weeks, we slept in our car or in Salvation Army rooms for free, learnt that the cheapest glass of milk could be bought at a bar, that the cheapest lunch was early, with the waiters in the restaurant before it opened, and that the cheapest bed and breakfasts were in villages outside of the city. Our old Ford rose to the occasion, as we traversed the continent and had the time of our lives. The Automobile Association in the UK had given us an itinerary which ensured we could see a great deal of Europe's cities, monuments, landscapes and delights. At the end of it, though, it was time to come home.

* * *

Returning to Bombay brought me back to earth with a thud. My very first hospital appointment was to a forty-bed facility in Malad. I would go there twice a week to attend to the Out-Patient Department (OPD) and Operation Theatre (OT). I would travel by train in the afternoon but at 1 p.m. in 1963, the only moving objects on the entire Malad platform were a few stray dogs and myself—a far cry from the crowds that choke seemingly every Mumbai railway platform today.

It was at about that time that my father referred to me a patient in his fifties with a huge inguinal hernia that almost reached halfway down to his knee—something that probably would not be seen today. I must have been starving for work to have accepted the case because it was an especially difficult one for a surgeon still cutting his milk teeth! The only mitigating factor was that, for a change, Dad had referred a well-off patient, who opted for a special room at the Prince Aly Khan Hospital and could afford the best medical care.

Although the surgery went off well, the patient did not pass stool or even a bubble of gas (flatus) for five days. While sluggish bowel activity was to be expected after operating on such a large hernia, a full five days without passing stool was stretching things a bit. Growing increasingly anxious, the patient and his relatives requested a second opinion. I asked them if they had someone in mind and, to my dismay, they asked for JJ Hospital's former senior surgeon whom I hadn't had the best experience of dealing with. I telephoned him, gave him the patient history and he agreed to come on the following terms:

1. I should be waiting at the hospital entrance at 10 a.m. to open his car door for him.
2. I should escort him to the patient's room.
3. On entering the room, I should give him his fees of 100 rupees (which I would take from the patient ahead of time).
4. I must follow his instructions to the letter.

I reached the hospital a little before 10 a.m., just in time for the doctor's car to arrive but not enough time to pay a visit to the patient beforehand. I opened the door for him to come out. He put one *chappal*-clad foot out, then waited to get his other foot out, ensuring that I held the door open for him. I led him up the stairs to the patient's room and, as he entered, whipped out a crisp 100-rupee note (given to me previously by the patient's relative) from my shirt pocket and put it in his extended hand for all to see. He stood by the patient's bed and said, 'Not even passed gas for over five days? There is obviously something wrong with the operation. Such cases must only be taken on by very experienced surgeons.' This declaration not only terrified the patient and his relatives, but me as well. He told the private nurse, 'Give him an enema immediately,' and was about to sit down, when the nurse replied in a high-pitched voice, 'Sir, he has passed a large stool with a lot of flatus this morning!' There was nothing more for him to do—the patient was on his way to recovery. He gave me a nasty look as he left, and I dutifully went after him to open his car door.

I never forgot this incident. At this early stage of my career, I was sure that no one would call upon me for a second opinion, but I swore to myself that if the opportunity ever presented itself, I would never ask the primary surgeon to be present when I went to see his patient, nor charge the patient any additional fees, nor criticize that surgeon in front of the patient, thereby respecting the primary surgeon's dignity. To my surprise, over the decades, I have been requested to give a second opinion both before and after surgery. And every time I give one, I remembered to make good my vow because the trauma of that incident in 1963 remains fresh to this day.

In the meantime, it was business as usual elsewhere. Professor P.K. Sen—for old time's sake, I suspect—had given me a part-time fellowship in the department of experimental surgery at the KEM Hospital (although he was miffed that I refused his offer of a full-time position as Assistant Professor of Surgery). Soon, I got appointed as the Assistant Honorary Surgeon at both the Bai Jerbai Wadia Children's Hospital and the JJ Hospital. Within a few months, I had resigned from the Malad hospital, and was enjoying the rich surgical work at the KEM, Wadia and JJ Hospitals.

The problem was that none of these hospitals paid for honorary work. For the first few years, my monthly income rarely reached four figures, but Khorshed and I had every reason to be satisfied with our circumstances. Surgery was my life, and I was getting plenty of experience. Khorshed's ambition was to keep a happy, cheerful home, and manage the children and the budget. We had a lot going for us. We lived rent-free in Nazir House in her parents' old apartment. Khorshed's father, in addition to the Parisian Dairy (an upmarket restaurant) on Marine Drive, owned a subsidiary of the restaurant in Fort, the business heart of Mumbai. Our lunches and dinners came from there—simple, nutritious meals. We were blessed.

I could perhaps have earned more, but I refused to capitulate to the culture of paid referrals. Khorshed and I were so used to the small monthly income and living on a shoestring budget, that we did not notice the slow but incremental increase in my income till we felt we needed to seek the services of an income tax consultant. There was no question about who our tax consultant would be—Dinshaw R. Bharucha, who was the tax consultant to both my father and my father-in-law. Dinshawji was a true-blue Parsee character. Scrupulously honest, he would not permit his client to hide a single rupee. On the other hand, he would not permit income tax commissioners to set terms either. The commissioners were afraid of Mr Bharucha. I am told by various people that he would barge into the income tax commissioner's office, slam his client's file on the table and ask how the income tax department had dared to question his client's returns. In all my years of practice, I have never had to pay a rupee to a single income tax commissioner under the table. He worked hard and late into the night, even though several of his clients were widows of his old clients whom he looked after free of charge, till the end of their lives.

My practice blossomed over the years, and money began to flow in, but I was and still remain clueless about managing money. At the end of each day, I would put all my money on the dressing table. I had no clue what I had earned that day, month, or year. Dinshawji would put an 'X' on the income tax form wherever my signatures were required. But through this rising income, I felt I learnt one of God's greatest truths—the less one chases or hankers after money, the easier, smoother and freer it comes.

Meanwhile, the family was growing. Ashad, our second son and third child, was born in 1964. Rushad and Ashad went to St Mary's, ISC. Dinaz started off in Walsingham, then followed in her mother's footsteps to Presentation Convent, Kodaikanal and for her last year, she went to Cathedral School.

In the late 60s, even though my practice was slowly picking up, I was afraid to leave work for even a day. During the children's school holidays in May and December, Khorshed would take them to Mahabaleshwar. I would take the night train to Poona every Friday, the first bus to Mahabaleshwar on Saturday morning, spend Saturday and Sunday with them, take the last bus to Poona on Sunday and the night train to Bombay, and be at work on Monday. At the end of the holidays, I would drive to Mahabaleshwar on a Saturday, and all of us would pack ourselves into our green Standard Herald MRY 7369 to come home.

In June of 1969, we were on our way home from Mahabaleshwar after the holidays in the car. The car was packed, there were two suitcases on the roof 'carrier', I was at the wheel, Khorshed was by my side, and the three kids were at the back. The rains had not started yet, but suddenly as we were approaching winding roads, there was a cloudburst. The road, covered with mud and slime, became slippery. I slowed to a crawl when a State Transport (ST) bus overtook us, cutting sharply in front of me, forcing me to slam the brake pedal. We slid across the road, and our car overturned, somersaulting into a ten-foot drop in a muddy field. We were extremely lucky, because there was a 200-foot drop on the other side into a valley. There was complete silence, and I was the first one to break it, 'Khorshed?' She replied, 'Rushad?' He replied, 'Dinaz?' No reply. 'Ashad?' Ashad replied. At least four of us were conscious.

Rushad was the first to act. The rear windscreen had fallen out. Rushad crawled out and opened my door. It was only after I got out that I realized the car had landed on its roof! Khorshed and Ashad were extricated from the car. Dinaz was conscious but stunned. I checked for injuries. Not a scratch on anyone, though Dinaz complained of a pain in the back of her neck. Rushad went into the car, got the camera from the glove compartment and we took pictures of the car upside down.

It was still raining and puddles were forming. Several villagers came to help, saw the car and could not believe that no one had been killed. Passing cars stopped to take pictures, sure of capturing fatalities, but did not stop to help, which was a reflection on our collective civic sense. The villagers brought long poles and turned the car back on its wheels. We took out sandwiches from the car and were enjoying a wet picnic, when we saw a small empty goods truck approaching. I waved it to a stop. The suitcases on the roof carrier, which had absorbed part of the impact of the fall, were put in the truck, into which all five of us crawled. The truck dropped us at the junction where the 'ghat' road met the Bombay–Goa highway. We arranged for a Jeep to take us to Bombay and a towing van to bring our faithful car back to us. The following day, we went to the Fire Temple to offer our thanks to the Almighty for our escape. Dinaz had a whiplash injury which settled in a few weeks.

As the years ticked by, Rushad got into medical college, and had no doubt he wanted to be a surgeon. I had the joy of working with him for twenty-five years on his return from England after his FRCS. He was a professor of surgery at JJ Hospital while being attached to the Breach Candy and Parsee General Hospitals. However, both he and his wife felt that their children, Farhad and Thea, would have a better future in Canada.

After passing the necessary qualifying exams, Rushad started his own surgical clinic in Vancouver. Their daughter, Thea, is now in her final year of law school at the University of British Columbia. Their son, Farhad, graduated as a doctor from the University of British Columbia, Vancouver and is now a resident surgeon specializing in vascular surgery. He represents the fourth generation of Udwadia doctors. My father would have been so proud.

Ashad followed in Rushad's footsteps and attended medical college too. After getting admission in 1982, he opted for orthopaedic surgery where he also met his future life partner, Reshma. After finishing their postgraduate exams, they married and left for England. Ashad did his Magister Chirurgiae (Orthopaedics) (MCh [Orth]) at Liverpool and has since been working as an orthopaedic surgeon at two hospitals in Greater Manchester. Their daughter, Simone, turned down admission to medical college to take up her childhood passion of veterinary surgery and their son, Rehan, more of an athlete than his father, was the Captain of Lancashire County Cricket Under 17s in the finals of the All England Under-17 Cricket Championship. He is now studying finance and business management at York University.

Dinaz opted to join HR College to study commerce. From among all my children, she was the one who inherited my sense of mischief, and always had a trick up her sleeve. Once, when Khorshed accompanied her to pay her college fees, she waited for what seemed like an eternity in the car, but Dinaz still hadn't returned. Parking the car, she went in to find out the reason for the delay. At first, all she could see was a long queue of students. Then, at the head of the queue, there was Dinaz, arguing with the clerk. Khorshed intervened, 'What is the problem? I am Dinaz's mother.' The clerk was on the verge of hysteria. 'You are her mother, and you ask what is the problem? On her college ID card, required to be shown to pay the college fees, she has got some boy's picture, and her name is given as Elvis Presley.' (Dinaz was an avid Presley fan). Khorshed, being her mother, told the clerk, 'Stop making a fuss over a silly prank and take her fees.' The clerk, who was now being heckled by the other students in the queue, could take it no more, 'The crazy girl has a crazy mother!' He got up, saying he was taking her ID card to the principal.

I was in a packed consulting room that evening when Khorshed phoned my direct line and asked me to come to

Dinaz's college immediately. 'Come to the top floor where Principal Dr Gidwani lives. Dinaz is about to be suspended, and Dr Gidwani wants to make a police case of forgery.' When I reached, my daughter was near the lift outside the principal's residence, while my wife was seated opposite Dr Gidwani, who was bristling with anger. Seeing me, he said, 'I am glad you could come. Your damn fool'—it seems 'damn fool' was Dr Gidwani's term for most students—'daughter has put my college in a precarious position.' Before I could ask how, he went on, 'Suppose she dies on the road and the police find her ID card with the college seal and her name as Elvis Presley, I would be charged with forgery, the damn fool girl!' I was about to ask why she should be found dead on the road, when I realized that that would be a damn fool approach. I had taken part in college dramatics. This was my cue. 'What!' I roared at the top of my voice, giving both Khorshed and Dr Gidwani a start. 'That is what that damn fool girl has done? I will take her home and give her such a thrashing. I will whip her with my leather belt. Tomorrow, you will see her black and blue from head to foot. No decent person can tolerate such behaviour. I will crush her!'

Dr Gidwani's face was ashen. He waved his arms in protest. 'No, no, no, Doctor, you cannot strike a girl! Please do not be violent with her, I will call her tomorrow to my office and scold her and confiscate the ID card. Call this damn fool girl.' 'Dinaz', I shouted and, when she entered, eyes appropriately downcast, aware of the act I was putting up, I asked, 'Why did you do this, you damn fool girl?' In a whisper, she replied, 'This boy had short hair and looked like Elvis, so I submitted his photo.' I raised my hand and went towards her as if to strike her. Dr Gidwani rushed to me, put his hand on my shoulder and said, 'Doctor, please be calm and control your anger; she is just a young girl.' We left Dr Gidwani's residence but not before hearing his final appeal, 'Doctor, you must promise me that you will not hurt her.' As we drove home, I wondered if my secretaries at my consulting rooms had been able to cope with the waiting patients as smoothly as I had handled Dinaz's near-expulsion in Dr Gidwani's office. Later though, as I got to know Dr Gidwani well, I realized he was an educationist par excellence.

After she graduated, Dinaz went to the Government Law College, Bombay to study law and complete her LLB. She usually had a full day. She would catch the early train from Grant Road to Churchgate, chatting with the fisherfolk on the train, finish law college at 11 a.m., go to Free Press House at Nariman Point, where she worked as a sub-editor for the *Free Press Journal* until 5.30 p.m. She would then come to my consulting rooms at 6 p.m. to help the secretaries. We would go home together after I finished my night visits. Her reward was that she could drive the car home. Her day did not end there, however. She would take dictation and type letters—a Brother typewriter having replaced the old Remington one by then.

Since 1985, Dinaz has been living in the United States with her husband Vispi, a Certified Public Accountant (CPA), who has his own private accountancy practice, and they both now live in Los Angeles. She subsequently graduated as a chef from the Cordon Bleu School of Culinary Arts, specializing in baking and pastry. Her daughter, Amy, a qualified hospital administrator, married Porus, an anaesthetist. Dinaz's son, Cyrus, is a vice president at Warner Bros.

In 2006, she was about to come to Bombay to see me receive an international award. The phone rang the day she was to leave LA and I happily asked, 'All set, Dinaz?' She started crying on the phone, 'Dad, I cannot come because I have cancer.' Shocked, I tried to comfort her while booking tickets for Khorshed and me for LA on the night of the award function. Dinaz, it seems, had a polyp (growth) in her uterus which was excised, and days later, the pathology report was a leiomyosarcoma. By the time we landed, Rushad and all our friends were already working on the best avenues of management. It was decided that an early radical hysterectomy was the way to go and to have it at Cedars-Sinai, LA under the care of Dr Beth Karlan. My mentor, Dr George Berci, was also at the same hospital. I met him with the request that he oversee Dinaz's treatment. George was in the OT throughout the operation, came out at the end and assured us all was well. Why my Dinaz? Why?

The wall of the waiting area at Cedars-Sinai outside the patients' rooms is made of glass. Every day that Dinaz was in hospital, I would stand in front of this glass wall and pray to God that she would forever be rid of this tumour, and that I would happily, willingly and gratefully take her sarcoma. Dinaz recovered, and all was forgotten. God in His infinite mercy held back His hand for eleven wonderful happy years of my professional and family life after which I was diagnosed with cancer for the second time.*

---

* Please refer to Chapter 6, The Surgeon as a Patient

2017 was the centenary of Einstein's discovery of the Theory of Relativity. The Einstein Foundation wished to celebrate the event by choosing '100 Visionaries of our Times' from all over the world. Surprisingly, I had been included in that list, and in June 2017, I had accepted the invitation to be in Montreal for a meeting of the 100 visionaries that October, and to deliver a talk there. The following month, we were in Manchester visiting our younger son, Ashad, and we planned to celebrate my birthday there. On 20 July, I was scheduled to meet Mrs Sybill Storz in Tuttlingen for an important meeting pertaining to the Center of Excellence for Minimal Access Surgery Training (ceMAST), a laparoscopic training centre for surgeons in Mumbai. Throughout my stay with Ashad and his warm family, I suffered from an unusual delay in my bowel habit, which did not respond to medication. I also felt some abdominal discomfort, which rang alarm bells. Colon cancer runs in my family and I had operated on my own father for it. I instinctively palpated the left side of my colon—because that's where I found the cancer in my father—and found nothing. But the next morning, after belatedly remembering that the colon is also on the other side, I palpated the right side to find a lump the size of a tennis ball.

While it is my habit to exercise caution, I had a knee-jerk reaction to the discovery and instinctively changed my travel plans, cancelled the meeting with Mrs Storz, and started making arrangements to return home. I telephoned my secretary Celina and confirmed that my onco-surgeon friend Dr Praful Desai was in Mumbai. We reached Mumbai on the eighteenth. Two days later, I had a CT scan with contrast at the Breach Candy Hospital, under the care of Dr Anirudh Kohli who headed the radiology department. While the mass turned out not to be colon cancer, it was confirmed to be a retroperitoneal mass, displacing the ureter (the tube connecting the kidney to the bladder) and adherent to the inferior vena cava (the large vein in the abdomen conveying blood to the heart).

Two days later, Anirudh did a CT controlled biopsy of the tumour. I went through the door connecting the CT room to the console room where the radiology team monitor all activity. When I saw the biopsy specimen—1–2 mm thin cylinders of white tissue like they had been removed from a pomfret—I knew what the diagnosis would be: retroperitoneal leiomyosarcoma. I booked Praful and Dr Sudhansu Bhattacharyya for the following week for my surgery. There were no symptoms that preceded it and fortunately, the cancer had not spread, but the vena cava had to be partially excised and grafted by Dr Bhattacharyya.

Intubated, on the ventilator for several days after the operation, my vocal cords could not function, and I lost my voice. Farokh put his heavy foot down and told me that I could not dream of going to Montreal after such a short time following the surgery. Dinaz was still in Bombay to help Khorshed look after me. With family support, an expert physiotherapist and monitored nutrition, my physical condition improved. But I still could not speak. Dr Milind Kirtane suggested speech therapy by Zainab Nagree. She came every day for speech therapy exercises, and Dinaz made me do them three times a day. I emailed my status—both physical and vocal—to Helen Haztis, my contact at the Einstein Foundation. She said the foundation would go to any lengths to ensure I could be in Montreal.

In October, I left for Montreal, although I could not make the full trip in one go. I had a three-day stopover in Zurich, one of Khorshed's and my favourite destinations. When we landed in Montreal, we were whisked away in a limo straight from our airplane to our hotel. I was doing my speech therapy till two hours before I was due to give the talk. My voice was clear, distinct and loud when I made my speech. Even after my surgery, God continued bestowing his kindness upon me.

3

My Mother

One of the biggest influences of my life, my mother, Perin, was the fourth of five children born to Pirojsha and Banoobai Lentin. My father came from a background so humble that he was forced to give up his dreams of studying further to become a surgeon, and start working immediately as a general practitioner to support his family. Pirojsha Lentin, by contrast, was a manager at Petit Mills and had built Banoo Manor comprising four-bedroom apartments in 1934. In 1939, my parents, Farokh and I moved into the ground floor apartment of Banoo Manor from our small apartment in Tardeo. My mother's parents moved to a new home constructed by her father called Château Marine, one of the first apartment buildings on Marine Drive. Before the Second World War started, Pirojsha Lentin had constructed ten houses in Bombay, among them Lentin House on the road connecting The Taj Mahal Hotel with the Radio Club, and Lentin Chambers, a large office block in the business hub of Bombay. Mummy did her schooling at the rigid Miss Moos School, popular with parents of Parsee girls at that time. She then went to St. Xavier's College, where she did her BA (Hons.).

Sports did not interest her; her great passion was the piano. She took her piano exams—certified by the Trinity College of Music, London—and had passed her Licentiate (LTCL) exam before she got married. She was preparing for the ultimate Fellowship (FTCL) exam after her marriage but had to skip it due to the birth of her first child, my brother Farokh. That did not, however, diminish her love for the piano. She continued to take lessons in three-month stretches, twice a year. Hearing her play 'Für Elise' was like listening to a recording by Artur Rubinstein himself. The piano in Banoo Manor was in the sitting room which had two doors, both opening into the garden. When she played for one hour every evening, passers-by would stop and listen.

Mummy married Daddy—Erach Udwadia—in 1929. It was a marriage of contrasting backgrounds. She had lived a more affluent life, mixing with other well-to-do Parsees and holidaying at their bungalows in Khandala at least twice a year. But from the day she married, she lived according to my father's means. For almost ten years, till we children were old enough, there were no trips to Khandala, and certainly no luxuries. Daddy would work from morning to night. His only 'outing' was going to Udwada to visit his retired parents and brother. He had set up a small general store across the street from their home to keep his father occupied. Daddy worked in the poorest part of Bombay—the mill districts of Lower Parel—and charged his patients considerately. He came home every night and put all his earnings in a tray on the dressing table in their bedroom. While it looked like he brought home a lot of money, the actual value was much less because most of his fees were in annas, not in rupees. That said, when Dad brought home two anna and eight anna coins, he did so with pride and satisfaction.

Each day's collection would be sorted, recorded and placed in a cardboard box to be banked at the end of the month. My brothers and I learnt a great deal from Mum. One of the most fundamental lessons she taught us was that the expenses must never exceed the income at any time. Another was that a hundred rupees earned through hard work and honesty were worth more than a thousand earned dishonestly.

We had a live-in cook and a part-time help to give Mum a hand with the housework. We boys were trained not to add to their workload and clean up after ourselves. Beds had to be made every morning, and books, clothes, shoes, toys and cricket bats, were to be kept in their appointed places. Mummy taught us that, like most matters, discipline starts with the small things.

Mum also imparted to us standards of honesty which went far beyond stealing or lying or not keeping your word. Her idea of honesty was to be true to oneself, to be honest from within, which had to manifest in all of one's activities. Her beliefs encompassed the fundamentals of the Zoroastrian religion— good thoughts, good words, good deeds—and its basic prayer (*Ashem Vohu*), which is to be righteous not in anticipation of future rewards, but for the sake of righteousness. She also believed we are what we are by an accident of birth and that we should look upon those who were less privileged with kindness and generosity.

I was the most difficult of her children and she was the most worried about my education. To her, a good education was the cornerstone of life. I used to play the fool and I was normally ranked in the top ten in my class. Her expectation was that we were all like Farokh and rank among the top three. Every month, she would walk to Gowalia Tank, an umbrella under her arm for sun or rain, get into the Number 10 tram, get down at Mazgaon and walk to our school to check with Father Molina, the principal, as well as with my class teacher about my academic performance and behaviour. She insisted that I read aloud while I studied, to make sure that I was not reading a story book from the class library.

Farokh was eight years older than my younger brother Darius, who was born in 1939, which is why I was far closer to Darius. Darius was quiet, a little nervous and, for a few weeks after he joined my school, needed me to hold his hand all through the long recess. Our longstanding relationship has only strengthened over the decades, and I can always count on him to be the first to stand by me in times of need. But I also felt he went a little overboard taking Mum's advice about studying aloud, and it was maddening when he read loudly for all his law exams.

Mummy had three brothers and a sister, but none of the brothers had any children. All of them were very fond of us and would occasionally call us over to spend Sundays with them. One such Sunday, Kekoo uncle and Homai aunty invited us over. Their dog had just had puppies and only one was left to be given away. I asked her if I could take him home. Farokh was not interested in dogs, and Darius was too young. She replied 'Of course, if Mummy is agreeable'. When Mum came to fetch us, she said yes. I was so excited and happy that I needed to pass urine urgently. I went into Kekoo uncle's toilet. There was a Western-style pot there which I had never used before as we only had one Indian-style toilet at home. I passed urine in the pot as best as I could. We took the puppy home in our car, fed him and we all went to sleep. We named him Bonnie.

In the morning, Bonnie was nowhere to be found. We frantically searched the entire neighbourhood. The cook thought he might have slipped away when the door was opened for the milkman. We were about to phone Homai aunty to confess and apologize that we lost the dog when a very angry Homai aunty phoned us instead. She was livid that I had not only urinated all over her toilet seat, which she had then sat on, but that we had deposited a small, defenceless puppy outside her apartment door without having the decency of ringing the bell. Mummy explained everything to her, including how we had been looking all over the neighbourhood for Bonnie since early that morning. How Bonnie, a newborn puppy, found his way back to his mother's home overnight on roads he had never walked on, remains a mystery to this day.

After a lot of pleading on my part, Homai aunty agreed to give Bonnie back to us. Bonnie was my dog, but all day when Mum was alone, he would follow her around and sit at her feet. Every night after everyone had gone to sleep, he would jump onto my bed and jump out before Mum came into our room. Mum or I would take him for his walks. I would pull out his ticks with Dad's forceps, drop them into an old Pond's bottle filled with kerosene and watch them die the moment the kerosene touched them. Every time I removed a set of ticks, Bonnie licked my face—the ticks must have been torturous for him. Bonnie was a part of the family, jumping all over Dad when he came home, trying to snatch the ball when we were playing cricket, lying near Mum most of the time. When he died, ten years later, Mum was in mourning. She cried, lost her appetite and stopped playing the piano for several days. Gradually, and to our relief, she came out of it. Mum had the softest, most loving heart of us all.

Till Dad's practice picked up, we would remain in Bombay during the summer holidays. When Mum felt we had the resources, we would take three-to-four-week vacations to places like Simla, Ooty, Kashmir and Ceylon. While we did not stay in luxurious hotels, they were memorable trips in their own way. I especially remember the Parsee-owned Blessington Hotel in Simla with fourteen rooms, six of which were occupied by Italian prisoners of war. We saw them in the dining room at mealtimes, after which they were escorted back to their rooms, where they remained confined all day. For us, holidays were not about luxury but a time for fun and stronger bonding with the family. I remember the time we stayed at the house of one of Daddy's patients, Mr Framroz Daruwalla, right in front of the sea in Golvad. It was a large family home with a big garden. Every morning after our baths, Dad call me to the veranda facing the sea and would teach me our Parsee prayers. There is one prayer in which a short sentence is repeated three times and Dad would say the prayer while banging his ruler on the marble table to a waltz beat. One morning, Mum caught Daddy doing so and got annoyed, 'Erach, you even make a joke out of our prayers!' Yet all the prayers I know and say every morning are what I learnt during that holiday. I haven't learnt any more prayers since then but have not forgotten a word of what Dad taught me.

To most mothers, their first child is their favourite, and so was the case with Mum, and not without good reason. Farokh was the model child, well-behaved, studious, clever, with no bizarre behaviour of the kind that got me suspended from school. Mummy, I felt, desperately wanted a girl after Farokh. That could be perhaps why she dressed me in a frock with my hair flowing down to my shoulders till I was three years old, and even got a picture taken; a picture my children find hilarious and still bring up in conversation. I still have this picture in my study. In her eyes, Farokh could never do any wrong. This did not upset me greatly, but little Darius felt the brunt of it, because he too was not a 'good' boy, and neither was Firdaus, who was sixteen years younger than Farokh.

By then, Dad's practice had grown. He also opened another dispensary at Dongri, which saw well-placed patients come in, mostly Aga Khani. Soon after Khorshed and I were married, she and Mummy were invited to lunch by the family of one of Dad's Aga Khani patients. It was a sumptuous meal, served sitting on carpets. Mum and Khorshed were made comfortable by being given big cushions to sit on. After the meal was over, a lady gave Mummy a glittering stone-inlaid bowl with a lid that opened with the help of a lever. Mum took some time to figure out how to open the lid, found the bowl clean and empty, and thought she was being given the bowl to appreciate it. She said, 'how lovely,' and was signalled to pass it to Khorshed. Khorshed opened it, hoping there would be chocolates inside but saw that it was empty and passed it to her neighbour to admire the bowl. The neighbour opened it, cleared her throat and spat a thick yellow large blob of sputum into the bowl. As it turned out, the bowl was actually a spittoon to be passed around and had been presented first to Mum and Khorshed as they were the guests of honour! We live and learn.

But before we got married, Khorshed was the biggest thorn in Mum's side. Mummy was convinced that she would be my downfall, my ruination. She based her view on what she concluded were undisputed facts. During the SSC exams, Khorshed had no contact with me, and I did very well. In my first year at Wilson College, I had been in contact with her, and nearly failed (in truth, this was because I was terrible at arithmetic). During my inter-science year, I was not in contact with her and I did well—my mother giving me no credit for studying hard and late into the night. Mummy was somewhat mollified by the fact that I did well in my final MBBS despite being in proper contact with Khorshed for almost two years.

After my MBBS, when I secured marks that ensured I would become a surgeon, I tried to convince Mum that Khorshed and I needed to get engaged because we had known each other for over seven years. She was reassured, but not enough to agree as Farokh had not yet been married! That is when Dad stepped in and convinced Mum that, instead of being a hindrance, Khorshed was a strong motivation for me to work harder. Mum, to my surprise and joy, finally relented. Once we were engaged, she became Khorshed's friend. She invited her home for lunch every Sunday. The Udwadia boys ate their food so fast, we would usually have finished before Khorshed had even picked up her knife and fork. Fortunately, Mum very frequently invited her nephew Bomi (later Justice Bakhtawar Lentin) for lunch too. If Khorshed was slow, Bomi was even slower, and we had to wait and 'follow the match' to see which of the two of them would win the slow-eating contest.

After Daddy passed away, Mum insisted on retaining her independence and maintaining her quality of life by herself. As an expression of her independence, she would drive her Premier Padmini—at best, she was a poor driver—onto Warden Road and, finding no parking space, would usually park in the middle of the road, as if her car was a divider. Many times, one of her children would pass by, see her car in the middle of the road, panic and hunt her down in nearby shops. For years, she lived all alone in a flat in Palacimo, a building constructed by her brother Minoo. Her long-time cook Lawrence retired to Goa and there was a part-time cleaning lady with whom she enjoyed a fierce daily quarrel. In her solitude, her piano was her best friend. These were the years when we were the closest. Palacimo was on my way to Breach Candy Hospital, where I worked, and I had told Ramu, my driver of over thirty-five years, that he should make sure I visit her twice a week. Ramu improved on this by making it three times a week, if possible. Without warning sometimes, he would turn the car towards the building and when questioned, had the same stock answer, 'Last time you were there for a very short time.'

If she was playing the piano when I got there, I would wait outside and listen to her with pride. Mum would act surprised to see me, but I was sure she had been hoping I would come. We would sit at the dining table, hold hands and talk. I would listen to her problems with stocks and shares (of which I understood nothing), her wanting to sack the cleaning lady (from which I would dissuade her), about missing her neighbours in the next flat (Rusi Cooper, his wife, Zarine, and daughters Phiroza and Farida, had all recently moved to Singapore), who, over the years, had become like her family and had looked after Mum and Dad with love. I would go to the kitchen, make two scrambled eggs with butter (she liked her eggs soft), toast with butter and hot coffee, and bring it on a tray to the table. She would say, '*Tehemton tey ai pachu kidhu*' (Tehemton, you have done it again). She would eat it with relish. After forty-five minutes or so, she would give me a hug and a kiss as I left. Once a week, I would get up on the piano stool to wind the wall clock. That clock was special to me; it had been bought by my grandparents during their holiday in Germany in 1934, on the day I was born. Mum would keep telling me how the clock was as old as I was! We would bring her home for lunch every Sunday, when Khorshed would make sure that her pleas of 'no more' were turned down. Did I do all this out of a sense of duty? Certainly not! I visited her as an infinitely minuscule token of my love for her and my gratitude for all she had done, sacrificed and devoted for the sake of her children.

Today, knowing the bitterness of a lonely day, I feel sad and ashamed that I did not visit her every day of the week. I rationed my time with her to just two days a week, with the kind and gentle Ramu often adding a third day. Was I so obsessed with work that my warped sense of priorities made me place a patient above my own mother? At the age of eighty-eight, I feel the neglect I showed towards my lonely mother more than ever, with a greater sense of shame. When she was mentally and physically unable to live alone, Farokh moved her to his house, where she lived for many years until she passed away. Mum's teachings and love live with all her children, and at times, when confronted with a difficult decision, I often ask myself, 'Would Mum approve?'

4

Four Hospitals

My surgical career could not have been possible without more than a little bit of luck. I was lucky to have trained where I did, at the time that I did, with the legends that I did. Four Hospitals pay homage to not only the wonderful people who guided and inspired me, but also to some of India's notable medical institutions.

Bai Jerbai Wadia Hospital for Children

At a time when institutions dedicated to paediatrics were scarce—across the world, not just in India—the Wadia Trust had the foresight to dedicate an entire hospital to both the medical and surgical care of children. Set up as an eighty-bed hospital in 1929, it was still an eighty-bed hospital when I did my surgical residency there in 1957. Over the past sixty-five years, the Bai Jerbai Wadia Hospital (or Wadia Hospital, for short) has grown into one of the world's leading paediatric hospitals in terms of volume, quality, innovation, training and research.

But to me, Wadia Hospital is special because of those who had a deep influence on the surgeon I am today. There were two paediatric surgery units headed by Major Rustom Irani and Dr Arthur D'Sa at the time, and the two chiefs could not have been more different. Irani, ramrod straight as befits an Army Major, had a stern smile and was a strict disciplinarian, but also principled, fair and correct. His surgical worldview was either black or white, with no room for grey. He took responsibility for every junior who worked with him, inspiring loyalty. He addressed every nurse as 'sweety' in the tone of either a 'sweet' sweety, a 'growling' sweety, or a 'get-off-your-ass' sweety. Without intending to cause offence, I picked up his habit and for decades, used this word. Of course, things have changed now, but it was useful when one worked with multiple teams across different hospitals and remembering new names seemed overwhelming.

Dr Arthur D'Sa, my guide during my MS at the KEM Hospital, was an entirely different kettle of fish. Handsome, debonair, smiling, outgoing, prone to giving a friendly slap on the back, he was the heartthrob of all the ladies at the hospital. An accomplished athlete, he was also part of the Lusitanian hockey team, which won the All India Hockey Championship regularly. A gifted and gentle surgeon, Arthur could teach surgery without a word, just by example. Wadia Hospital was a homely place and at lunchtime, Arthur would drive across from KEM with his lunchbox on his operation days, frequently humming or singing his favourite Goan songs. At KEM Hospital picnics, he needed little persuasion to roll up his trousers (most people didn't wear shorts at that time) and burst into a Goan song-and-dance routine. On one occasion, when I was a consultant, I went to Arthur for advice on how to deal with the severe criticism of my work in laparoscopy. His reply was, 'Tehemton, they are critical because they did not think of it first. Believe in what you are doing. Don't give a duck's fuck about what they say.' This piece of advice is something I have passed on to all my residents.

The assistant paediatric surgeon at both units at Wadia was the gracious Dr Charles Pinto, whom we called Charlie, and who went on to become one of India's leading paediatric plastic surgeons. The chief of the orthopaedic paediatric surgery unit was Dr Rustom Katrak, now known as the 'father of Indian orthopaedic surgery', who was extremely learned, yet simple and self-effacing.

And then there were my colleagues: Dr Subhash Dalal, the registrar from whom I learnt not only the fundamentals of my surgical craft but, and more importantly, the niceties of surgical behaviour. And I cannot forget the contributions of Shantu Vaidya, the resident anaesthetist, who grew into an innovative plastic surgeon, and taught me the value of simple joys. He also taught me that friends are forever. He bought twelve plants for the resident quarters at the hospital and after evening ward rounds, we would take a 'plant' round to admire them.

There was also Hirjee, Farokh's best friend from St Mary's school and KEM Hospital, who was also the son of Wadia Hospital Superintendent Dr S. Adenwalla. Hirjee and I were also good friends, bonding as we did over our common interests in surgery and cricket. Hirjee lived on the Wadia Hospital premises and was always ready to lend a helping hand. After his MS, fulfilling his quirky Parsee desire to follow in the humanitarian footsteps of Dr Albert Schweitzer, he got a job at the Jubilee Mission Hospital in Trichur, a nine-bed facility where he was surgeon, physician, gynaecologist, anaesthetist et al. He taught his wife Gulnar, fresh out of school, to work in the ward and the OT, and built a full-fledged team from scratch. Together, his team transformed a dilapidated nine-bed facility into a teaching hospital that is now a world-renowned centre for the surgery of craniofacial deformities and crippling birth defects, that were genetically transmitted and endemic to the Trichur area.

While Hirjee had access to basic medical care in this specialty, having worked with Charles Pinto at Wadia, he invited him to Trichur and, between the two of them, they set up the internationally renowned The Charles Pinto Centre for Cleft lip, Palate and Craniofacial Anomalies., which to this day trains surgeons from all over the world. As part of the team behind the Smile Train (for the surgery of the cleft lip and palate), Hirjee continued operating well into his nineties and was a living testament to how one person's integrity, passion and foresight could move mountains.

Tata Memorial Cancer Hospital

The Taj Mahal in Agra is rightfully one of India's contributions to the wonders of the world. It has stood for centuries, majestic, being visited by hordes of tourists from all over the globe. I, however, feel that the Tata Memorial Cancer Hospital (TMH) has equal right to be considered one of the wonders of the world. Consider a typical day at TMH—it is difficult to enter the hospital, for every entrance is choked with patients entering or exiting. Caught in the current of patients and relatives pushing and squeezing their way in the vague direction of their destinations, it could take over an hour to reach where one needs to go. Corridors, passages, halls, and stairwells are similarly packed with patients from every part of India and beyond. While the contrast between the TMH and the Taj Mahal could not be sharper, the right of both to be considered wonders of the world could not be more equal.

In 1958, I worked at TMH as a resident surgeon. Over the years, I visited frequently on invitation as a consultant, but on 2 January 2022, I was there as a patient, accompanied by my son Rushad, now a surgeon in Vancouver. On 3 January 2022, which was a Monday, Rushad and I met Dr George, the Head of Thoracic Surgery, at 10 a.m. to check my investigations. A soft-spoken, gentle and smiling man, Dr George made it seem like I was the primary reason he had come to TMH that day and gave me all the time in the world.

Nothing could move until I was registered as a patient and my TMH file was made. A resident doctor in his Tata garments was deputed to make a path for Rushad and me, akin to an icebreaker ship in the Arctic. He elbowed his way through to get to the registration office at a little past 11 a.m. My file was made, my photo taken and the receipt for the hospital deposit submitted. When I was being handed my file, I was told to always remember my file number—1050. That means that from 1 January to 3 January (when I got my file), 1049 patients had been registered before me. Between Saturday, a holiday on Sunday, and 11 a.m. on Monday, when I was registered, two amazing things struck me about this—the number of patients and the capacity of the facility to diligently register them. This in itself, according to me, was a miracle.

At TMH, there is no time or space for pleasantries and superficial courtesies, but every patient—most of them poor and destitute, and many of whom spend the night on the pavements outside the hospital when the doors are finally closed—is treated with respect and dignity. This enormous load is shouldered by a team of unquestionably dedicated staff who seemed to enjoy the daily onslaught of patients, almost to the point of masochism. Standing outside the consultant's office, one wonders if the staff would be able complete the day's load even by allotting one minute per patient, but magically, they always do. And every patient leaves satisfied with their consultation. How do they manage this day in and day out? What fuels their devotion?

The evening after my procedure, performed by Dr S. Kulkarni, Head of Interventional Radiology, Dr George came to look me up on his way home. I wanted to give him time to reach home before I called to thank him again for his kindness, but an unfamiliar voice had answered the phone instead. 'I am sorry, Sir. Dr George is scrubbed for an emergency and will not be free for a while.' It was back to business as usual at Tata Memorial Hospital. Wonders are made on earth; miracles are made in heaven.

The infrastructure at TMH is stretched to the utmost but continues to deliver with passion and efficiency. Tata Memorial Hospitals have now been set up across the country, and rightly so, because the demand is far too great for one centre to meet. If the patients can't come to TMH, the logical solution is to take TMH to the patients.

P.D. Hinduja Hospital

It was thanks to the efforts of Dr Noshir Wadia, the internationally renowned neurologist, and his future wife Piroja, whom I interacted with at JJ Hospital for my surgery and research, that I was appointed as a consultant surgeon at Jaslok Hospital, which was conveniently located within walking distance from my residence. A year later, on a matter of principle, I walked into the CEO's office, stood in front of him, asked for a piece of paper, and wrote out my resignation letter with a sense of relief.

I do not know if it was an accident or if there was a grapevine between hospitals, but the very next afternoon, I got a phone call from Hinduja Hospital saying that the CEO would be happy if I went to meet him the next day at 2 p.m., as he wanted to consult with me about a conference the hospital was hosting. I went to Hinduja Hospital the next day but was told that the CEO's office was at Hinduja House in Worli, and had to rush to keep my appointment.

I met the CEO, a paediatrician from the US, who was in temporary command at the time and whom I never saw again. I asked how I could help with the conference. He took a long pause and then startled me by saying, 'Dr Udwadia, the Hinduja Hospital would like to invite you to join as Consultant Visiting Surgeon.' No manna from heaven could have had better timing or be more appreciated. As the expression goes, you could have knocked me over with a feather!

I joined Hinduja in 1987 and for over thirty years, I experienced almost the same pride, satisfaction, joy and atmosphere of compassion that I had at JJ. While the workload was only second to JJ, it was a small part of the reason for my devotion to the hospital. Hinduja was spotlessly clean, disciplined and above all, ethical—no unnecessary hanky-panky referrals, courteous and accommodating colleagues, no shortcuts in patient care, and no cuts to speak of!

For over thirty years, I devoted every Friday to Hinduja Hospital, and it was for me, a day of utter joy—OPD in the morning, OT for the rest of the day and then rush to my consulting rooms at Cooks Building, Fort. Dr Santhi Swaroop Vege, Head of Medical Gastroenterology at TMH was also the head of gastroenterology at Hinduja. He would refer the surfeit of patients waiting interminably for surgery at TMH to Hinduja. Hence, added to my load of general surgery, there was the responsibility of onco-surgery. While it was hard, backbreaking work, I called upon my residency training at TMH thirty years back in 1957 to tackle its unique challenges.

Three months into my consultancy, the matriarch of the hospital, Lalitaben Hinduja, invited me to her office on the first floor of the hospital for tea. We clicked like two magnets. She was the soul of the hospital. She knew every employee on a first-name basis. She taught me how to deal and interact with all kinds of people, from the dignitaries who visited from Massachusetts General Hospital (affiliated to Hinduja) to the lady who cleaned the hospital washrooms. She would take a round every day, and it was always a great learning experience for me to accompany her. Adding to the joy of working at Hinduja was the pleasure of collaborating with the resident staff. Every registrar here had cleared their MS exam, and was highly experienced, so interacting with them was a great learning experience for me. Later, I also benefitted from the support of the senior residents who were Diplomate of National Board (DNB) fellows, each one as sharp and keen as a razor blade. After Dr Deepraj Bhandarkar and Dr Avinash Katara came on board as consultants to supplement my efforts, the quality and tempo of my work increased greatly with their excellence.

One incident was particularly unforgettable. On Fridays, it was routine for me to rush to my consulting rooms at Cook's Building after finishing my surgical cases in the OT at Hinduja, but as it happened, I was running late that day. The last case was a colonic resection (excising the tumour in the colon and re-joining the two cut ends). We started at 5 p.m. and completed the anastomosis (joining the two ends of the colon) by 6.30 p.m. As my consulting room had already started at 5.30 p.m., I left immediately after the anastomosis. I was at the elevator waiting to go down when I was summoned back to the OT—there was a complication that needed correction. I scrubbed in again, and after completing the re-anastomosis, I left. It would take me thirty minutes to reach my rooms now making me well over two hours late. There were no mobile phones at the time, so I requested an OT nurse to phone my secretary, and ask her to send away as many patients as possible.

Every Friday evening, my devoted driver Ramu would keep a paper cone of *chana sing* ready for me, put an Air India pillow on the back seat of our Premier Padmini car, cover me with a small, soft Air India blanket, and rush me to the office while I slept. I dreaded going to my consultancy rooms so late and hoped that most of the patients had been sent home. Keval, the liftman at Cook's whose duty was over at 6 p.m., but who never left until I went home (no one had heard of the word 'overtime' back then!) saw me and said, '*Aaj kuch gadbad hai*' (there seems to be some commotion). I opened the door and I felt as if I was stuck to the ground. Expecting to be confronted with sullen and angry faces, I was dumbfounded at what I saw. The two secretaries, Celina and Pervin, had converted the long wait into a picnic. Patients were chatting, laughing, and eating samosas and vada paos. As soon as I entered, I was invited to join the party! The clinic ended after 10.30 p.m. on a happy note. The two secretaries had turned the situation on its head, converting the angst and annoyance of the patients into happy acceptance. These two ladies, along with my first secretary Mani Treasuriwala, worked with me for decades, and were worth their weight in gold. Sloppy and ill-disciplined as I was, I could not have survived without them.

After Lalitaben passed away, I had pleasant interactions with S.P. Hinduja and his daughter Vinooji, as well as Mrs Usha Raheja (daughter of Lalitaben) as also all the brothers, especially Ashok. The family has always treated me with kindness and tolerance, a thirty-three-year bond of joy and performance.

Dr R.N. Cooper and the Dr R. N. Cooper Municipal Teaching Hospital

There is always a reason a hospital is named as it is, and the story behind it has always intrigued me. A hospital could be named after a country like the All India Institute of Medical

Sciences (AIIMS), after a city like the London Hospital, after royalty like King Edward VII Memorial Hospital (KEM), or a leader, like the Indira Gandhi Hospital. They could also indicate their location like the Great Ormond Street Children's Hospital or the generosity of a philanthropist like The Johns Hopkins Hospital, which was named after a banker who made the largest-ever single donation in the United States at the time.

There is, however, one hospital in Mumbai that does not subscribe to the usual conventions. The Dr R.N. Cooper Teaching Hospital is not commemorative of any donor, corporate house, royalty or family. It is named after a gentle and self-effacing surgeon who passed away decades before the institution was named after him. I can safely say that Dr R.N. Cooper was a legend in his time, the mentor of all mentors, on whose guiding principles the foundation of Indian surgery rests today.

In a country where the naming of every bylane, chowk, or gully becomes a subject of heated debate and is often politicized, it is remarkable that a teaching hospital in Mumbai was named after a simple surgeon by the Brihanmumbai Municipal Corporation (BMC) with unanimous consent. The original R.N. Cooper Hospital, a modest hospital in Juhu, Mumbai, was affiliated to and given teaching status as a part of the KEM Hospital in 1977 and was upgraded to the current Dr R.N. Cooper Teaching Hospital in 2015 with 940 teaching beds and an annual intake of 200 medical students. The Directorate of Medical Education and Research (DMER) granted the hospital permission for affiliation to the Maharashtra University of Health Sciences, Nashik.

But what was so special about this surgeon? Dr R.N. Cooper was the first Indian surgeon to obtain the MS (London) and the FRCS (England). Upon his return to India, he was refused an appointment at the JJ Hospital, his alma mater, because he was not British. Their loss, however, was the newly founded KEM's gain, where he was immediately appointed as Honorary Surgeon and Head of the Department of Surgery. He was also made the honorary director of the Bai Jerbai Wadia Hospital for Children.

During a safari in Kenya, I was informed that a group or a family of magnificent royal lions, the majesty of the animal world, was termed a 'pride' of lions. Dr Cooper and his contemporaries at KEM were certainly a 'pride' of surgeons.

There was the surgeon with an 'Einstein mind', Dr Ramchandra Ginde, whose financial situation was so precarious that Dr Cooper had to personally ensure his survival. Blood transfusions, routine today, were then elaborate procedures that were conducted in operating theatres and required senior supervision. By requesting Dr Ginde to attend to all the blood transfusions of his patients, Dr Cooper helped keep him financially afloat. Dr Ginde went on to become one of the founders of neurosurgery in India, an international figure. He was manic about precision, and he remembered every single patient he had ever touched. Later in life, though, I dreaded meeting him on the golf course as he would voluntarily and enthusiastically keep correcting my grip and stance, till I could not tell if I was on the golf course or his resident doctor being reprimanded!

Then there was Dr A.V. Baliga, my mentor, who, because he could not get an acceptable matriculation certificate in

India, overcame all odds to do his London matriculation, then the Licentiate of the Royal College of Physicians (LRCP), Membership of the Royal College of Surgeons (MRCS), and finally, the FRCS to become the master surgeon of India in his time.

Dr G.M. Phadke helped bring urology to India, and introduced the Millin's operation, a different method of removing the prostate. A gruff, physically imposing figure, his bedside clinics were a draw, and he had a habit of rubbing his thumb against the forefinger as he taught. I was once told off by him for I forget what, but I do remember him saying, 'You . . . you . . . you so called son of your . . . your . . . your so-called . . . so-called father, you . . . you . . . don't know this simple thing?'

Another dominant member of the pride was the legendary surgeon and my mentor, Dr Prafulla Kumar (P.K.) Sen with whom I worked for over a decade in surgery and surgical research, and who made me who I am. Unlike most Indian surgeons who trained in England, Sen trained in the United States and was convinced that training in experimental surgery was the only way to make a surgeon complete, a belief that he passed on to me. With a view to ultimately work on human heart transplants, he conducted an experimental surgery project on dog heart transplants, for which Sharad Pandey and I were on the donor side, and Dr G.B. Parulekar and he operated the recipient's end. Later, on 16 February 1968, he performed the fourth heart transplant in the world, putting KEM and Indian surgery on the global map.

Dr Vasant Sheth was yet another special surgeon. I don't know if he ever possessed a watch, but he never needed one.

'I will take the next class at 2.30 *saarp*.' He would come at 5 p.m., the exact time his consulting room would start. He would take the lecture till 7 and leave us with the words 'next class at 2.30 saarp.' In the 1950s and 60s, suicide attempts were unfortunately quite common among impoverished wives in the Parel area of Mumbai, and the widespread method was to drink pure sulphuric acid. While they often survived, their oesophagus would be destroyed and would need reconstruction. Few had the ability, patience or time for this difficult and lengthy operation, but Dr Vasant Sheth did. The operation would go on and on.

At the time, in addition to assisting with the operation, it was mandatory for the registrar to be with the patient all night, so using creative ways to find a short reprieve was often necessary. William Samarji, Sheth's registrar, would tell me at breakfast that he needed 'help', which meant that he needed a break during the operation, so that he could pull through the night shift. Halfway through the procedure, I would dutifully scrub, enter the theatre, and tell Dr Sheth, 'Sir, I will replace Samarji for a while as he is urgently required to be a witness in a murder case.'

I enjoyed assisting Dr Sheth—every move was stated aloud, the reasons given, and the consequences of improper procedure detailed, which he would describe in gory detail. I am quite sure he talked in his sleep. After a patient underwent a long procedure under the anaesthesia available at the time, he would visit the patient in the middle of that night to check on the post-operative status.

Then, of course, there was Dr R.N. Cooper himself, the Lion King. He had retired as head of surgery long before I joined

GS Medical College in 1951, but had continued taking classes for postgraduate students as Emeritus Professor of Surgery at KEM. I never missed his class. A friend of my father's, he was very concerned about the welfare of the students, and he knew that for the last six months of our final term, with work and study, we were very short on time. He would come well before his lecture, write his points, make his colour drawings (he was good at making diagrams), so that our time would not be wasted seeing him write and draw on the board. His little snippets, in between topics, like 'there is no minor surgery, only minor surgeons', or 'humility is the essence of a master surgeon', were lessons that have stayed with us forever. Always forward-looking and encouraging of talent, the last thing he said at the end of his last class with my batch was, 'My greatest joy and pride is that my students and residents are doing bigger and better surgery than I have done.'

Dr Sunil Pandya, the neurosurgeon who followed Dr Homi Dastur as the Head of Neurosurgery at KEM Hospital, once told me about a few of his experiences with Dr Cooper. While a student at Grant Medical College (GMC), Sunil was interested in the history of medicine. Being aware of Dr Cooper's passion for the subject, he wrote to him to ask if he could study from some of the books in his vast library. Almost by return post, Sunil received a kind letter inviting him to meet Dr Cooper at his clinic. The Lion King received him courteously, complimenting him on his interest. Sunil requested if he could come once a week, take a book from the library, and read it on the balcony of the clinic. Dr Cooper replied that it would be an inconvenient way of working and that Sunil should take two or three books home at a time, then come to return them and take more. We must remember that he had never met this young student before, who was from a different college. To this day, Sunil remains amazed and humbled by Dr Cooper's trust in him, a total stranger, to handle such precious books.

On another occasion, Dr Cooper was called in by Sunil to examine a patient with an abdominal crush injury who had developed kidney failure. He told him that he had just got a book on surgical advances in which this problem was discussed. He felt patient management needed to start immediately, and asked Sunil to phone him at his residence at 9 p.m. Over the call, Dr Cooper painstakingly and carefully read out the entire chapter so that Sunil could understand and make notes and start treatment immediately. Involvement, empathy, care, passion and action were his core values.

Dr Cooper showed me immense kindness after I returned from England. I was appointed Assistant Honorary Surgeon to the Wadia Hospital when he was the honorary principal medical officer. At the Association of Surgeons of India (ASI) conference in Delhi, the year before the Silver Jubilee Conference in Mumbai, he hosted a dinner for several senior surgeons. As Khorshed and I could not afford to stay at a Delhi hotel, we stayed at the Parsee Dharamshala, where we paid a princely sum of seven rupees for stay, breakfast and dinner. He sent a car to take us to his hotel for the function, where I turned purple with embarrassment when he introduced me, a complete unknown, to some of India's best senior surgeons as 'Tomorrow's Surgeon!'

Dr Cooper started his long career at the KEM with the creation of a department of surgery that ranked among the best in the world for the period between 1930–1970, during which I was at different times a student, a resident and a fellow. The only member of the ASI to be made president of the association twice, Dr Cooper was universally referred to as 'Daddy Cooper' on the KEM campus. And while every nurse to Major Rustom Irani was 'sweety', every student or resident to R.N. Cooper was 'sonny'. Just as I picked up 'sweety' from Major Irani, I picked up 'sonny' from Dr Cooper and continue to use these terms. About ten to fifteen years ago, Ramya, a DNB fellow at Hinduja, was blessed with twins. The day after the delivery, I visited the twins and asked him when he would name them. He replied, 'I have named them after you.' 'After me?!' I cried. 'Yes! The boy is named "Sonny" and the girl is named "Sweety"!'

Decades later, the powers that be at the Medical Council of India (MCI) and the University of Mumbai, deputed me to inspect the R.N. Cooper Hospital, to help them decide if it was ready to be recognized as a teaching hospital. I found the staff keen and capable, the teaching programmes good, and the infrastructure adequate. I was clear that the hospital merited the elevation, and I submitted my recommendations accordingly. My decision, in any case, was a no-brainer. Any hospital with the name of R.N. Cooper attached to it had to be fit to be a teaching hospital.

Unlike surgeons from other teaching hospitals who proclaimed, 'we are the greatest', the mantra of the KEM's pride of lions was always 'we need to get better'. That said, any reference to those giants cannot be made without mentioning their empathy and generosity in giving of themselves as honorary surgeons. I am convinced that the glory of Indian medical teaching was during the honorary system. These highly qualified doctors and surgeons spent the better part of their working day (morning to noon) teaching students and treating poor patients with total dedication. They did this for free, often brought their own equipment, and remained available for overnight emergencies. Their service was an expression of their love and duty, and they cheerfully worked extra hours later in the day to compensate for the hours they spent at teaching hospitals. This was not only in Mumbai—it was the universal Indian medical teaching culture of the time. Honorary appointments were difficult to get—only one would be chosen from several applicants. I was blessed to be given the opportunity to work as an honorary surgeon at the JJ Hospital for thirty-two years of my career. What I learnt is priceless. The honorary medical system of education has given us most of today's leading medical consultants in every branch of medicine.

5

The ceMAST Story

While my ward 19A at the JJ Hospital had a capacity of twenty-five beds, we usually found ourselves attending to forty to sixty patients at any given time. There were patients on the beds, on the mattresses, on the floor between beds, under the beds, in the corridors, in the passages—all of which pointed to a serious lack of infrastructure and diagnostic facilities. My senior colleague, Dr Rasik Patel, and I would wrack our brains to find ways of reducing the backlog and hastening bed turnover.

In December 1971, I was waiting outside the OT at Breach Candy Hospital, about to go into surgery. Normally, the anaesthetist, Dr Gulab Bhagat, would be in the OT before me, but, on this occasion, he was delayed. Fidgeting, I peeped into the adjacent theatre and saw Dr Nargesh Motashaw* conducting a procedure with one eye peering into a telescope. I asked her what she was doing, and she replied that she was doing a laparoscopy. I had never heard that word before. I asked her what laparoscopy was and she invited me to have a look. I scrubbed and put my eye to the telescope. I was

---

* The name was misspelled in the earlier book.

flabbergasted by what I saw. The entire pelvis was illuminated, with perfect anatomy, colouring and presentation. I requested Dr Motashaw if she could reverse the table tilt. She readily agreed and when the head end was raised, I saw the liver, the stomach, the duodenum, the gallbladder, the spleen, the colon, the bowel, the diaphragm, omentum and the entire abdominal anatomy, just as I would have seen during an open surgery. Moreover, the view was complete with magnification, perfect light and vision! It immediately struck me that this was the ideal method of diagnosing patients who came to us with abdominal symptoms. Maybe this would be a quicker way of increasing our bed turnover! I have always thanked Dr Bhagat for coming late that day—because his delay literally opened a whole new horizon for me—and Dr Motashaw for my first view through a laparoscope.

After getting the details of the equipment, I wrote to Karl Storz, the manufacturer of the equipment in Germany. In those days, the import duty for medical equipment was so prohibitive that it was cheaper for Khorshed and I to go to Germany, buy the equipment, and bring it back ourselves. In February 1972, Khorshed and I drove from Frankfurt to Tuttlingen in a red Japanese car—the cheapest and smallest we could rent. When we arrived, we were shown to the office of Mr Storz. He was a six-foot-four, big-built, stern-looking man. Since, at that time, no surgeon was using a laparoscope, he took it upon himself to show me the equipment. He had set out the entire range required for diagnostic laparoscopy and explained the workings of the first and the simplest instrument, the Veress Needle. Like any true Indian, the first question I asked him was how much the Veress Needle cost. When he told me, I started haggling. 'It's too much for a simple needle!' I told him. 'Surely, you can reduce the price?'

Mr Storz wouldn't budge. 'Professor Udwadia, fixed price always at Storz,' he replied curtly. And so it went on. With every new piece of equipment he showed me, I would ask the price and request a reduction, and he would say the same thing, 'Fixed price always at Storz.' He was getting increasingly irritated, and when we finally came to the telescope, he snapped, 'If you want it, you pay for it!'

Presently, it was time for lunch. Probably feeling that I didn't have much money, he offered to take us out for a meal at a nearby restaurant. As we were walking through the parking area, he stopped in front of my small red car and shouted, 'This is not possible, this cannot happen in Germany! A Japaneeese car in Germany?!' I said it was the only car I could afford to hire. He looked at me as though I was something the cat had dragged in. During lunch, he spoke only to Khorshed.

On the walk back, he told me, 'You, a surgeon, want to buy a laparoscope, when you know nothing about laparoscopy? I will show you some movies made by the gynaecologist Dr Kurt Semm (pronounced Zemm) so that you understand what a laparoscope is and how it is to be used.'

When we got to the office, he said, 'You are fortunate, we have got a new 16 mm film projector.' At that time, most teaching films were shot on 16 mm film and loading them on the projector was quite a cumbersome process. As the film was taking time to load, I walked over to take a look. When the loading was over, I said in a very harsh, loud voice, 'Mr Karl

Storz, this is not possible, this cannot happen in Germany, a Japaneeese projector in Germany!' The projector was a Fuji!

Mr Storz turned red with anger, got up and walked over to me. As his large frame bore down on my relatively smaller one, it struck me that I wouldn't need the red car to go back to Frankfurt—I would be going back in an ambulance. Suddenly, Mr Storz burst out laughing. He laughed and laughed, and between the Japanese car and the Japanese projector, we forged a friendship with him and the entire Storz family, that has lasted for fifty years now. He did not reduce the price of equipment, though!

While I have always had a good relationship with the Storz family—starting in 1972 with the founder, Mr Karl Storz, and latterly with his grandson, Karl-Christian—my longest association was with Mr Storz's daughter, Mrs Sybill Storz, from 1982 to 2021. I would meet her at all ASI conferences and several international endoscopy conferences. She would seek my opinion on current and future trends of laparoscopy and when laparoscopic cholecystectomy burst on the global scene, I was put on the priority list for the supply of equipment, despite there being a long queue of impatient surgeons the world over.

In 2005, she was an integral part of a unique, 'model' three-year public-private partnership between Storz and the government of Germany for a project on maternal care in northeast India—where maternal mortality rates were the highest. As per her request, I was part of the study and the final report at the conclusion of the project. When I eventually met her after that, I asked how a private company had been able to match the financial input of a state government. She replied that Storz was a family-owned company, with no shareholders to answer to, so she could spend her profits on causes of her choice. It was then that I requested her to set up a laparoscopy training centre in India, although I didn't specify the city.

I thought our conversation would not go anywhere, but in 2011, after Europe had recovered from the financial crisis of the previous three years, she asked me to meet her at an international conference where she told me she was ready to start a laparoscopy training centre in Mumbai with me as Chairman. She had two conditions, though—firstly, no live animals were to be used, and secondly, its purpose was to be solely training with no commercial activity. I was delighted to accept her terms, but I had two conditions of my own—that Dr Gadgil, who ran the Johnson & Johnson (J&J) training centre in Mumbai, would be made the director, and that the centre would be an autonomous body run by surgeons for surgeons. She agreed. And so ceMAST (the Center of Excellence for Minimal Access Surgery Training) was born, with no MOUs or documents, but just a handshake.

Dr Gadgil brought in Parag Mulay, a true Man Friday, into the team, and with Pradeep Ajmera, Mrs Storz's personal representative for Storz in India—who, for over forty years, had helped set up Storz in India—we settled for an area of 4,000 square feet opposite Mahalaxmi Racecourse. Brijesh Chinai was appointed as the architect with Jamshed Shaikh working alongside him. We would meet onsite every week to keep track of the project.

The centre opened on 22 July 2002—a gleaming, state-of-the-art facility with two training laboratories, one tissue preparation room, one lecture hall that could seat forty people, a cafeteria, a registration area, and office chambers for all of us. The first to be recruited was Megha Patil, who manned the front office, and while she ultimately worked as my secretary, she was a great asset for ceMAST in general. We started with only three courses—general laparoscopic surgery, laparoscopic urology and laparoscopic gynaecology. The first course had a grand total of three participants, the second had four and the third, three. I was miserable, wondering if I had unwittingly led Mrs Storz into a financial debacle. I wrote to her with my misgivings, but she wound up consoling *me* by saying this was how all ventures began. She was right—over the ensuing months, the courses started to fill to capacity and over the years, the number of courses increased from three to sixteen.

The first chief guest at ceMAST was the President of India Dr A.P.J. Abdul Kalam. He had great enthusiasm for anything scientific or pathbreaking, both of which the centre was. He gave a stimulating address and followed it up with trying his hand at using 3D laparoscopic equipment. He was so involved with seeing the equipment in use and interacting with the surgeons, that his security team had to literally force him away as his airplane was holding up other flights at the airport.

ceMAST had several features that made it unique—faculty handpicked from all over the country both for their expertise and their love of teaching, as well as pig cadaver models for laparoscopic training that were designed by Dr Gadgil and the lab team to 'mimic' actual operative situations. These models included kidneys that were designed to 'bleed' during a partial nephrectomy, lungs that would 'breathe' or have foreign bodies or tumours implanted in the bronchial tree, and myomas implanted in the uterus.

Mrs Storz and her son Karl-Christian visited the centre and impressed with our work, she suggested that we move the training centre to larger premises. Pradeep Ajmera zeroed in on an office space in the Worli area of Mumbai that was three times larger than the Mahalaxmi centre. And while Mrs Storz was initially concerned about the financial implications of a higher rent, a larger staff and greater equipment requirements, she eventually greenlit the new ceMAST. Having visited training centres in several parts of the world, I knew that we could make this a world-class, one-of-its-kind centre. And we did. No centre in the world had either the passion for excellence or animal models even close to ours.

We were fortunate to have a reliable tissue and animal supplier in Mr Tambe, who would deliver these at the designated time without fail. A few pig cadavers were always stored in the giant deep freeze at -25°C as backup. Designed by Brijesh Chinai once again, the new, larger centre was accredited by various associations and societies, both national and international. Mrs Storz and her son came for the grand opening ceremony in the newly designed seventy-five-seater auditorium.

The ceMAST team, led by Dr Gadgil, also created a third ventricle with human anatomy in a brain model that would 'pulsate', the first of its kind in the world. Noted neurosurgeon and faculty member, Dr Deopujari, took this model all over the world, popularizing it and with it, ceMAST. After Dr Gadgil retired in 2019, Dr Suchitra Bindoria was appointed Director in his place, with Ms. Shikha Rudraraju in-charge of promotion and sales. I took over some of Dr Gadgil's work and, with the inputs of the lab technicians, created pig anatomy models for colon and liver resections.

My interactions with Mrs Storz went way beyond ceMAST. She often sought my views on future developments and focus areas in minimal access surgery and then factored them into her company's strategy. However, sadly, our relationship with the office of Karl Storz India (KSI) in New Delhi began deteriorating over time for reasons I found difficult to fathom. They perhaps wanted a say in the day-to-day running of ceMAST, but we were committed to keeping it autonomous. Then, on a visit to the centre in December 2019, Mr Diwakar Rana, Managing Director of KSI, casually mentioned to Dr Bindoria and me over a cup of tea that ceMAST would be shut down in a matter of weeks. The words were uttered so lightly that I hardly picked them up, but Dr Bindoria exclaimed, 'What!'

I emailed Mrs Storz immediately, but for the first time in our decades-long relationship, I got no response. I also telephoned her, but she was not available. It was then that I read the writing on the wall. Stepping down from the chairmanship of ceMAST was not an issue for me at all. After all, I had worked there for ten years, was well into my 80s, and in poor health. But I was heartbroken that a training facility recognized as one of the best in the world, and found worthy of affiliation by bodies like the Royal College of Surgeons of England, would be destroyed. However, thankfully, KSI decided to temporarily retain the staff of ceMAST, including Dr Bindoria as Director.

Dr Bindoria swung into action and, with her negotiation skills, initiated talks with Sun Pharma to take over the centre—talks that went on for months. Firmly believing in our vision of disseminating matchless medical training in India, the company readily agreed to take on the financial responsibility of running the centre. Thus, from the ashes of ceMAST, like a phoenix, rose the Institute of Medical and Minimal Access Surgery Training (IMMAST), supported by Sun Pharma.

I am convinced that the decision to appoint Dr Bindoria as Director of ceMAST was the most important one I took as its chairman. With her still very much at the helm, as the head of IMMAST, and no longer restricted to using only Storz equipment, IMMAST has expanded into training not only for MAS but also for cardiologists, pulmonologists and intensivists. With her remarkable thought process and commendable market research, Dr Bindoria has planned and launched courses in specialized medicine, hair transplantation, dental implants, treating the diabetic foot, and minor surgery for General Practitioners—a popular course which runs packed—among others. Sun Pharma appointed me as Advisor to IMMAST, even though Dr Bindoria does not need advice from anyone. I enjoy going to discuss current and future courses with Dr Bindoria and Dr Nikhil Patel, who oversees the creation of amazing new models for every new course.

One of my primary beliefs in life is that whatever God does, is for the best. The closure of ceMAST, for whatever reasons, turned out to be a blessing in disguise. ceMAST was but a shadow of this new training facility, which owes its success to the vision of Dr Bindoria and the farsightedness of Sun Pharma. IMMAST is continually evolving to offer courses not thought of by any other training centre across the world.

6

The Surgeon as a Patient

When patients are wheeled in for surgery, surgeons often don't see what the patients see. They see a human form draped in a unisex gown, hair tied back under a cap, body parts shaved as needed and skin scrubbed clean with antiseptics. They see the area to be operated upon, which is usually marked and draped in sterile towels. They see a case—complete with charts, readings and histories. They see a challenge—a puzzle to be solved, discovered, or investigated. They see an opportunity— to relieve pain, to heal, to cure. What they see is different from what a patient sees.

For the patient, the surgery could represent a culmination of months or years of discomfort, of ignored symptoms, of suffering. The operation may have created a fresh set of problems—financial, emotional and professional. On the night of admission, on an unfamiliar bed, in a strange room, they may have been woken up by staff assigned to monitor their vital signs—the first of many interruptions. They may be alone, or with their kin, fielding anxious calls from family or friends. They try to stay, or are kept, upbeat but even their surgeons can't always predict the outcome.

They are awoken at an unearthly hour, prepped and wheeled by masked strangers into the OT. Often their first experience of being operated upon, most patients are usually terrified, surrounded by more masked people moving around silently. Their anxiety intensifies as another unfamiliar person, the anaesthetist, introduces himself or herself. Standing around the patient are nurses, technicians and assistant doctors waiting for the anaesthesia to kick in. In the meanwhile, the patient's only familiar link to the operation, their surgeon, is yet to make an appearance. Where is the surgeon? You can usually find him or her waiting for the anaesthesia to take effect or having a cup of tea between cases or in the ward to see a patient or attending to a call in Casualty. By the time he or she enters the OT, the stage is set, and the patient is 'under'. This process is routine for everyone except for the patient.

Today, the bond between surgeons and patients has weakened to such an extent that surgeons often cannot see, let alone feel their patients. The time when patients need them the most, is when they are entering the operation theatre. If patients were to see the encouraging face of their surgeon—perhaps the only familiar one in the room—it could significantly defuse their fear of the unknown.

I am deeply convinced that every surgeon should go through the ordeal of being draped in a unisex OT gown, lying on the operation table surrounded by masked strangers, looking around anxiously for their surgeon to make an appearance as they slip into anaesthesia. It is my firm belief that this experience would make them kinder and more sensitive to their patients' anxieties.

I must be a very slow learner, for the Almighty found it necessary for me to go through the experience of lying on the OT table several times. Each operative procedure I have undergone has been a wonderful learning experience that has influenced the way I approach surgery and patient care.

My first surgery was the outcome of a condition that was first observed when I was at Wilson College. Professor Wagh, my NCC Platoon Commander, noticed that my left little finger was bent, during a platoon inspection. He asked me to straighten it out, but I couldn't. As it didn't bother me in any way, I ignored it until it was noticed again years later by Narain Chhabria, when I was working with him as a research fellow in Professor Sen's unit. The flexion deformity of my left little finger had increased with time and after showing it to Dr Sen, who mistook it for leprosy, I subsequently went to the orthopaedic head, Dr K.T. Dholakia (KTD), who correctly diagnosed it as a 'recurrent anterior dislocation of the ulnar nerve with some nerve thickening and damage'.

In my case, every time I flexed my elbow, the ulnar nerve crept over the protrusion in the ulna bone, and this repeated dislocation of the nerve over the ulnar bone had been damaging the nerve over time. It had to be fixed, else it would come in the way of my performing surgeries later in my career. What KTD planned to do was to transfer the nerve from behind the bone and fix it in the front of the ulna, so it would not be repeatedly bruised every time I flexed my elbow.

I could not afford a nursing home but was happy to be admitted, at no cost, in the hospital I worked at (KEM) with my friends near me. The night before the surgery, I got my

93

first taste of being on the 'other side'. Alone, in a small side room of the orthopaedic ward, I worried about Khorshed. We had been married for just eight months and she was four months pregnant. If something untoward happened to me during anaesthesia or surgery, what would she do? I was bordering on a state of panic till I took hold of myself and reminded myself that my anaesthetist Dr Ambardekar, besides being a friend—we had played cricket together for years—was wonderful at his job. And Dr Dholakia was the best in his field. I could assuage my anxiety because I knew the quality of my team, which is a kind of 'insider information' that most anxious patients don't have access to. As expected, the procedure went well, though I still have a permanent claw deformity of my left little finger, which has not progressed after surgery.

I believe that the memory of the deep panic I felt that night, at the very beginning of my surgical career, has made me a better surgeon. Care of the patient begins well before the operation, and handling its emotional and psychological trauma is as much a part of the surgeon's remit as the surgery itself. For over six decades, I have visited every patient the night before surgery to reassure them and advised a good, mildly sedated, night's sleep. The next morning, before I operate, I briefly remove my mask (much to the nurses' annoyance!), hold the patient's hand and ask them to think happy thoughts as they go under. The anaesthetist is instructed not to begin the case unless I am present in the theatre. As someone who has experienced general anaesthesia, I have often likened the feeling to entering death. Patients don't know what is going to happen; they'll be clueless, unconscious. And it's the fear of the unknown which it is the surgeon's duty to dissipate.

As it turns out, the ulnar nerve operation was only the first of many and more serious procedures I was fated to undergo in my lifetime. In 1980, I developed severe back pain that I initially attributed to golf. Thinking it would go away with time, I didn't give it much importance until an incident where I was operating. At that time, there were no hand switches for the cautery machine, and we had to use a footswitch. During one surgery, I could not tell where my foot was. In the middle of the operation, I realized that I had lost my kinaesthetic (awareness of place and position in the body) sense. I completed the procedure by standing on my heel with the footpad just in front of my toes, in a way that I did not have to move my foot. I then knew that I had a major problem, and it had to be resolved.

The tests eventually revealed that there was pressure on my spine that was causing my back and foot problems. At that time, spine surgery was still in its infancy in Bombay, and Dr Gajender Singh, Dr Bhagwati, and Dr Dholakia were the ones who had just started doing it. Reluctant to operate on my problem, they asked me to wait for an American specialist, Dr Cloward from Hawaii, who often came to India to see spine patients. At about the same time, it seemed that JRD Tata had also developed a spine problem for which he was advised surgery. The Tata team went on a hunt for the best spine surgeon, and finalized Dr Patrick O'Leary in New York. When I was playing golf one day, JRD Tata, who knew about my problem, kindly suggested that I should consult Patrick myself.

During a call with him, I felt as if Dr Cloward was uninterested in my illness. On the other hand, my phone conversation with Patrick O'Leary was more about my surgery and vague about the fees. I preferred the latter because of his attitude, and of course, due to the fact that JRD himself had recommended him. I fixed the surgery for mid-September 1985 in New York. As senior surgeon to Air India, I, and by association, Khorshed were entitled to first-class travel, which of course I did not complain about. At that time, Air India's First Class was the ultimate in air travel.

Patrick admitted me to a renowned hospital in Manhattan. My radiologist turned out to be a former student at JJ Hospital, Dr Patel, who recognized me and did not bill me for his services, which I thought was extremely kind. At the time of admission, I had requested for a double room, which in itself was stretching my budget, but Dr O'Leary shifted me to a special private room at no extra charge.

While Patrick was as warm if not warmer than an Indian surgeon, the nurses who tended to me were an altogether different story. My interactions with them were unpleasant, to say the least—at one point, I was even given another patient's medication! They made us feel that common Indians like us had no business occupying the same hospital rooms as CEOs and royalty. When Khorshed mentioned this to Dr O'Leary, he replied that there was precious little he could do as the issue fell under the hospital administration's domain, and he had little to no say.

Patrick expertly removed the pressure on my spine, which relieved me of the back and leg issues. As somewhat indicated during our first telephone conversation, he did not charge me his fees. At that time, there was no ban on the export of ivory; so, as a thank you, we had carried with us an exquisite ivory piece of a fisherman to gift to him when he called us over to his Park Avenue home. He loved it and placed it on the grand piano in his sitting room (a standard feature of all Park Avenue apartments, it would seem). He would work at his two hospitals five days of the week, clear all his paperwork on Saturday and spend Sunday doing charitable work at churches and church schools. He was a true Irishman transplanted to Park Avenue. Khorshed and I continue to maintain our warm relationship with him to this day.

From Patrick, I learnt the warmth of a colleague from a different culture and from my experience there, I was able to fully appreciate the true value of Indian nurses, who are gentle, kind, courteous and efficient, always willing to go the extra mile for the patient. While rude and inefficient nurses are pampered in other cultures, our nurses are often treated with scant respect. This injustice needs to be corrected and their wonderful qualities need to be recognized.

* * *

The following years were relatively quiet on the surgery front, barring one for a right inguinal hernia, which was thanks to my sudden enthusiasm for lifting weights at the age of sixty-five. My son Rushad, who did an excellent hernia repair, operated on me so smoothly that I was able to check on my patients on my way back home from the hospital.

In 2004, when I was about seventy, I noticed a small lump less than a centimetre in size in the right side of my neck. True to form, I ignored it until I was asked by Dr D. Pahlajani, a cardiologist, to get a thallium test done to check my heart. While the heart was normal, Dr Lele, who performed the test, informed me of the presence of a small neck nodule which had been picked up by the dye. I showed the test results to Dr Praful Desai, who fixed a procedure at the Parsee General Hospital for a right lobe thyroidectomy with frozen section (the lesion was sent for histopathology while I was still under anaesthesia). As I was being induced by Dr Bhagat, Rushad was holding my hand. Praful gently moved him aside, gave my palm a squeeze and said, 'no worries, Tehem', as I went under. The frozen section was malignant, reported as a papillary carcinoma and Praful very rightly performed a total thyroidectomy.

After the operation, and after I had had some time to recover, the endocrinologist suggested that I test to see if there was any distal spread of the malignancy. When Khorshed and I went to pick up the report, I was also informed that I had multiple lymph nodes in my neck and chest and immediately needed to be admitted to the nuclear unit at Hinduja to destroy the malignancy in all the nodes. While I was surprised to hear this, Khorshed was devastated. I dropped her home, while reassuring her in the car, and went to meet Praful to inform him of the developments.

Praful told me not to worry about the nodes in the neck, because they were probably a reaction to the surgery. The CT scans had picked up the nodes alright, but they were not part of a malignant process. The dependence on technology is so heavy that today's surgeons will send the patient for a CT scan without even a physical examination, and then use the scan to tell the patient what is wrong with them. I took Praful's advice, and I have had no thyroid issues for almost twenty years.

It would be a while before I would be in the hospital on a personal matter again, but I could never have imagined that the next time was going to be for an emergency concerning my older brother Farokh. We were on holiday with my daughter Dinaz and her family in Los Angeles when I received a frantic call from Praful that Farokh was seriously ill. He was in hospital and had had no bowel activity for days. Praful was being pressurized by other consultants to operate and investigate, but he was convinced that doing so would cause Farokh grievous harm. Farokh had asked for second opinions, and had received many, but Praful told him the only opinion that he would accept as his doctor, would be mine.

I immediately cut short my holiday, wondering on the flight back how—after decades of acrimony between us—Farokh would accept my examining him. But the moment I saw him on the bed, my heart flipped. He appeared anxious and vulnerable. It was at that moment that regret started coursing through my veins. I cursed myself for not having built bridges sooner between us. He was my best friend for the first two decades of my life and we should have remained close to each other. I stroked his cheek; he gave me a familiar smile. I asked if I could examine him.

Those who know Farokh as a physician or a colleague, know that he is a brilliant clinician. I was sure he would have already diagnosed his own illness, which he said was caused by mistakenly eating tinned oysters that were past their expiry date. While most were sceptical about this never-before-heard diagnosis, I knew he was right. I also knew that that would mean the condition would be self-limited and timebound. I totally agreed with Praful that to open and mess around in an abdomen with a lethargic, paralysed bowel (as a result of the oyster toxin), would be a futile and dangerous exercise. Praful was visibly relieved to hear me say it. I reasoned with Farokh that the only treatment was a combination of patience, nutrition and the symptomatic treatment of the distention.

Inactivity was alien to Farokh's nature and he insisted on numerous tests. Most had been done before I came, including a colonoscopy, a diagnostic laparoscopy, and several radiology procedures including a Barium study, all of which had been inconclusive. Gradually, over the course of several days, the intestine resumed functioning, spasmodically and segmentally, till full function was finally restored and Farokh was well. God could not have designed a better way to bring us back together. Farokh gifted me a silver Zarathustra, which has pride of place in my dining room.

When it was my turn next, Farokh repaid me many times over. In 2017, Khorshed and I were visiting Ashad and his family in Manchester for my birthday. Throughout my stay with him, I had an abnormal delay in my bowel habit, which was not responding to medication. Lying in bed one night, I remembered that at about this age, my father had colon cancer on his left side, which I operated upon. I palpated the left side of my colon, but didn't find anything, forgetting that the colon is on the right side as well! Next morning, I realized my oversight, and felt a large lump the size of a tennis ball.

I usually take my time to respond to things, and am not prone to knee-jerk reactions, but I instinctively knew that I needed to return home, and I brought our travel dates forward. On my return, the CT scan showed that the lump was not colon cancer but a retroperitoneal mass, that was displacing the ureter (tube connecting the kidney to the bladder) and adherent to the inferior vena cava (the large vein in the abdomen conveying blood to the heart). I already knew my biopsy report when I saw the biopsy specimen—what was removed from my body was 1–2 mm thin cylinders of white tissue that looked like they were shredded from a pomfret. It was a retroperitoneal leiomyosarcoma, which was involving the vena cava.

Retroperitoneal leiomyosarcoma is a dreaded form of cancer with very few survivors. The only hope of a few years' survival is provided by a total resection of the tumour. Praful agreed to perform the surgery. I requested Praful if Dr Raman Deshpande could assist him and insisted that Dr Sudhansu Bhattacharyya (Bhatta) be the cardiovascular surgeon along with his anaesthetist. Bhatta would need to graft-repair the vena cava if he found that the vena cava was involved, but it was a high-risk procedure.

As predicted, Praful mobilized the entire tumour expertly, and found it was indeed adherent to the vena cava. Bhatta removed a wedge of my vena cava and sutured a gortex graft to restore continuity. Resecting the vena cava at this stage caused my blood pressure to drop. However, Bhatta's anaesthetist Dr (Mrs) Mhatre expertly restored my parameters. Bhatta is a magician, and the credit goes yet again to our common mentor, Professor P.K. Sen.

After the operation, I was in the ICU on a ventilator. When you're lying in bed on a ventilator, mucus and pus can collect in the lungs, which can cause a lung infection, a major post-operative complication. To prevent that, every few hours, a physiotherapist would come in, whether I was asleep or awake, thump my chest, and play a heavy tabla piece on it for about twenty minutes to dislodge any obstruction in the small bronchi and keep the lung clean.

For almost ten days after surgery, I had not passed a bubble of gas or a teaspoon of stool and was grossly bloated, distended and on the verge of being both delirious and septicaemic. I realized how easy it was to hallucinate when one was very ill. While, in reality, the ICU room was small and rectangular, I had visions of being in a palatial room with balconies above where physiotherapists were looking down at me and discussing what *raag* to play next on my tabla. The duty room outside looked like a large foyer with people passing by in formal clothes. The commode wheeled regularly into the room looked like it was a pot from hell, which was odd because the steel seat was freezing cold.

Two people were constantly by my side throughout my surgery and the stormy postoperative period that followed—my son, Rushad, and my brother, Farokh; what was gratifying was my rapprochement with Farokh after decades. Both Rushad and Farokh took rooms in the hospital to attend to me during the nights throughout my seventeen-day stay in the ICU. One of my problems was the insertion of a Ryle's tube (which is a tube inserted into the stomach to suck out its contents and keep it empty), which for some inexplicable reason, could not be passed into my stomach. On about the tenth postoperative night, unable to sleep, I was lying in bed, talking to Rushad, when suddenly, I hiccoughed and felt something slimy in my mouth. I spat it out—it was liquid faecal matter. I asked for a Ryle's tube and Rushad agreed that we should pass it into my stomach. The ICU registrar protested; they had tried to do this several times and failed. Rushad lubricated the tube with an anaesthetic jelly and gave me half a glass of water to sip as the tube went down. Within less than a minute, Rushad had passed the tube into my stomach, while I was sitting. Almost two litres of feculent fluid were aspirated from my stomach. From that moment on, I knew I would recover and endured the tabla played on my chest without complaint.

Praful would see me twice a day, and Farokh would spend long sessions in my room checking my reports and ordering new tests. Rushad was in and out, taking up the job of a gatekeeper, as no one was allowed to enter my ICU room, and provided regular updates to Khorshed, Dinaz, Ashad and my brother, Darius, who kept vigil in the waiting area outside the ICU all day, till late in the evening. I think they had a far harder time sitting outside the ICU than I had inside my room.

Even when I was moved out of the ICU and into another room, visitors were restricted. While they couldn't enter, much-loved visitors like Biki Oberoi and Reena Baruha, who flew over from Delhi just to talk to me for two minutes from outside the door, as well as others, like Mugat Shah, Subhash Dalal and Gulab Bhagat, made special efforts to lift my spirits.

I went home about three weeks after surgery. Rushad and Ashad eventually returned to their homes, and Dinaz stayed behind to give Khorshed a hand. I resumed work at ceMAST within two weeks of being discharged. It had been three weeks of holiday and about five weeks of surgery and recovery, and there was a lot of work to do.

* * *

The next few years went by, but clearly, my body had not had enough of surgery. When laparoscopy started, little attention was given to ergonomics with respect to the surgeon's comfort and the prevention of back and joint pain. After thirty years of laparoscopy, I developed problems with my shoulder, and an MRI confirmed there was gross arthritis with the destruction of the rotator cuff. While Khorshed was convinced that golf was responsible for this, I did a shoulder arthroplasty under the gentle and impeccable hands of Dr Dinshaw Pardiwala, who treats India's leading sportspeople. A left inguinal hernia was later repaired by Dr Ramesh Punjani, a colleague of mine who I saw evolve into an excellent and internationally recognized herniologist. Other surgeries included those related to a port placement for starting chemotherapy and a total knee replacement (TKR) of the left knee by Dr Sanjay Agarwala of Hinduja Hospital. As luck would have it, the COVID lockdown started the day after my surgery, ensuring all my physiotherapy was self-taught from YouTube!

In 2020, I discovered that I had multiple small bilateral lung metastases (spread of the tumour to the lung) before my shoulder replacement surgery, but I was not prepared to let cancer interfere with my quality of life, nor stop me from the surgeries for the hernia and the knee. That said, one particular metastasis in the right lung was abutting the aorta and the heart, and was growing at an alarming rate. This was ablated in a five-hour procedure that required both infinite patience and precision by the interventional radiology team at the Tata Memorial Hospital. The same lesion grew rapidly again, and was once more ablated by Dr S. Kulkarni at Tata Memorial Hospital in 2022. I have now been informed by the doctors at the hospital that there is no further treatment available to me.

I have learnt a great deal from each surgery I have undergone. During my surgeons' visits, I felt I owed it to them to reassure and comfort them that I am doing well. It also reminded me that there is nothing 'small' in postoperative care; a simple Ryle's tube not positioned in the stomach could have been a disaster for me. It is also best to avoid complaints about nurses or other staff as this creates negative energy, and is often counterproductive. But, most importantly, each episode taught me how essential it is to have total faith and confidence in your doctors and support staff, to be as cooperative as possible as a patient, follow all advice to the letter, and keep a positive outlook.

7

The Patient with Cancer

Cancer has inspired fear since centuries and most people fear cancer more than any other disease. The mere mention of it evokes associations of doom, relentless suffering, drastic treatment, pain, uncertainty, recurrence and death. The entire social system has given the darkest and gloomiest presentations of this condition, which is not always justified in today's scenario, where several types of malignancy can be arrested, contained and kept in remission, creating a new and vast generation of cancer survivors. While there are many illnesses more lethal than cancer, it is on a positive yet realistic note that I present the true impact and facts of being a cancer patient. I speak from personal experience.

Cancer is not one disease. It is an umbrella term covering a large number of diseases of variable venom and intensity. Yet all these numerous manifestations of cancer share one fundamental commonality—the growth of abnormal human cells which multiply with abnormal rapidity and spread locally and distally. Cancer has flourished for millennia, greatly dreaded and poorly understood. Even the excellent Pulitzer Prize-winning lifework of Siddhartha Mukherjee chronicling the biology of cancer from antiquity to recent times carries the factual but terror-inspiring title *The Emperor of All Maladies.*[*]

It is against this bleak and preconceived background that cancer enters the life of a patient. The patient may have some premonition of the possibility of the disease, or it may come as a bolt from the blue. In either case, when the patient visits the doctor, they must take one or more close family members for this once-in-a-lifetime visit. To receive a confirmed diagnosis of cancer impacts the individual heavily, causing physical, emotional, and psychological disturbance which requires immediate family support and sharing. The intensity of this impact can be greatly cushioned by the doctor conveying the news.

The delivery of a diagnosis of cancer is difficult by any standards. No patient likes to hear it and no doctor likes to say it. This moment is also a test of the doctor's honesty, empathy, experience and wisdom, for he bears the pain and sorrow of a message which will change the patient's life forever. The doctor needs to employ openness to explain to the patient and their family in simple words, the nature of the particular cancer— presenting it in favourable terms, avoiding the gory details at least at the first meeting. He must take the time to make the diagnosis understandable to lay people, and give ample time for the information to sink in, and then permit the patient and family to ask questions.

As a surgeon with a special interest in onco-surgery, I have been in a similar position to give advice and anticipate

---

[*] Siddhartha Mukherjee, *The Emperor of All Maladies* (London: Fourth Estate, 2017).

commonly asked questions. 'How dangerous is my cancer?' With my stock answer, 'Not as dangerous as crossing the road in Mumbai,' I explain the diagnosis in lay terms and stress that investigations are required to fully assess the situation. 'Will the treatment cure it?' The aim of treatment is to suppress the cancer and keep it suppressed for the rest of the patient's life. 'Can it recur?' Recurrence is the greatest anxiety for a patient. Perhaps, but with good response to treatment, it is unlikely to, and if it does, it can be similarly treated. 'Will the cancer kill me?' Perhaps, but that is again unlikely with treatment. While no one can call cancer a 'blessing', it is far better to have cancer than several other illnesses like terminal cardiac, renal or pulmonary failure, where there is continuous and often traumatic treatment to maintain a basic quality of life, and where the curtain can drop at any moment. The patient with cancer is on a comparatively better wicket, so count your blessings!

The first meeting is not the appropriate time to tell the patient how to cope with their cancer—that comes later. Despite all that is said, the patient will leave the meeting confused, anxious and angry, asking 'Why me?' Over time, realization will crystallize and the capacity to cope will depend largely on how the patient *accepts* the diagnosis, the degree of family support, and the guidance of the medical team. But I must emphasize here that the best results are seen in those who are optimistic, have faith in the treatment, the surgeon, the oncologist and who work together as a team to treat the disease, wherein everyone does their part, including the patient.

As the patient progresses on the journey with cancer, there will be other traumatic events—investigations, surgery, chemotherapy and radiation. All carry the fear of pain, deformity, side-effects and complications. Surgery is the oldest and most preferred mode of treatment while chemotherapy and radiotherapy are viewed negatively, as they are continued over time and unlike surgery, are used only for cancer. After treatment, there comes a period of tranquillity, if not peace, if there is no further evidence of disease. This phase permits a semblance of normal life, and as this disease-free period continues, the complacency and strength from being a cancer survivor seeps in.

But for some patients, there will be recurrence, which is the return of disease after a disease-free period, which can take from months to decades. Recurrence impacts both the patient and the family as much, if not more than the first diagnosis of cancer. Pessimism, feelings of injustice, questioning the value of the treatment, fears of death predominate. The resumption of treatment must be faced yet again.

I had been operated for thyroid cancer in 2004. For almost two decades, I have been free of the disease, foolishly believing that I had been cured, until one of my best friends, my golf partner Ashok, informed me that his wife Connie, who had been operated upon for a thyroid malignancy thirty years ago, had recently developed extensive recurrence of the same cancer. She was wonderful, brave and composed, and stoically underwent repeated surgeries. I would visit her after my rounds late evening at Breach Candy Hospital to comfort her, but would instead leave consoled and strengthened by her brave and philosophical acceptance of her progressive decline. When she was home, I would occasionally drop by to have a glass of wine with her and Ashok, and learnt how their acceptance of the disease ensured a peaceful and happy conversation through the evening. This taught me that while for thirty years, one may feel one is cured of cancer, but the fact is that one must continue as just a cancer survivor. It also taught me that acceptance of cancer is the essence of physical, mental and emotional peace for both the patient and their family.

The patient, thank God, does not go through this long, traumatic journey alone. The family accompanies the patient all the way. The feelings of distress in a loved one so threatened, are compounded as their own lives change when they take on the mantle of caregivers. Chemotherapy, physiotherapy, follow-up appointments, nutrition, physical activity, emotional tranquillity, hygiene, and the possible development of depression, need supervision and bring many changes to the lives of loved ones, too—these can disrupt their daily lives for a prolonged and unknown period of time. My wife Khorshed seemingly coped well, keeping her emotions bottled up until the bubble burst. She stopped eating, talking, going out, watching TV; all she did was pray and sleep. It took some time to bring her back to normalcy. Cancer can hit the family as hard as it does the patient.

Finally, if the cancer wins, there is the terminal illness. Death provokes the fear of the unknown in most people. Pain, suffering, loss of both dignity and of a sense of belonging are part of this period. Pain must be alleviated at all costs. On the subject of pain relief, one of the stupidest sentences I have ever heard a doctor say is, 'Surely, you will make him an opium addict!' It is a blessing being an opium addict for the last few weeks of terminal cancer! Today, there are pain management specialists who play a pivotal role in providing solutions devoid of opiates. At this stage, the doctor's involved presence and support in making the patient's life as comfortable as possible is an essential part of his duty.

Let us come to and remain with the happy ending: cancer survivors—those who have been treated for cancer and continue to live. More than any other time in the history of the disease, the number of cancer survivors is increasing exponentially now, signalling a significant shift in the battle against cancer, and providing proof that there is a stronger, happier light at the end of the tunnel. While they often bear mental and physical scars of the treatment, cancer survivors resume normal life with the passage of time, and face the future with hope and anticipation once again. Several survivor groups have been formed to guide, help and motivate survivors to learn to live joyfully, accept the life changes imposed by the condition, and make their peace with the disease, however temporarily. The dark and devastating picture of cancer as depicted to the lay public even today, needs to be revisited and redrawn to a more accurate and positive presentation.

To the patient with cancer, statistics don't comfort the patient—even if the incidence of a particular cancer within a population is low, it still affects the patient 100%. Hence, to give the full picture, I have supplied above a grim, depressing progress of cancer in the patient's life. But the forecast for the disease is not always gloomy. In fact, the clouds are beginning to part, and we can see rays of hope. I have been a surgical student of cancer from 1957 till today and have observed the journey of the disease closely over the last sixty-five years. We have come a long way from the time when surgery was extensive, radical, super-radical, supra-radical, horrifying and mutilating, to today, when we realize that extensive surgery mutilates and does not eradicate, and should be restricted as much as possible. This would validate the prophecy made three centuries back by John Hunter who said, 'This last part of surgery, namely, operations, is a reflection on the healing art; it is a tacit acknowledgement of the insufficiency of surgery. It is like an armed savage who attempts to get that by force which a civilized man would get by stratagem.'*

In the 1950s, chemotherapy was limited to nitrogen mustard, which was almost as lethal as the disease itself, sometimes hastening death. Now, the immense volume and quality of research that is ongoing in the war against cancer has given outstanding results in the treatment and suppression of some hitherto fatal forms of the disease, and the relatively effective suppression of innumerable other malignancies. Incredibly advanced, pin-point accurate radiotherapy, gene-therapy, immunotherapy and similar modalities are breaching the defence of cancer. Research into the future may be totally non-invasive, where nanos (much smaller than the size of an atom) will be injected into the patient and specifically programmed to destroy cancer cells!

---

* Maurice B. Strauss, *Familiar Medical Quotations* (Boston: Little, Brown and Company, 1968).

The key to coping with cancer successfully is *acceptance.* Several patients, on their own or with guidance, have found their own strategy which enables them to view cancer certainly not as a friend, but as an entity that has entered their lives, one they must learn to live with, for better or for worse. Several methods help, including surrounding oneself with positive and happy people, counting your blessings, focusing on your passions (golf is mine!) and celebrating your wins, whatever they might be. Accept the cancer in your body as an unwanted and unavoidable feature of your life, and also understand that acceptance cannot be attained overnight—it requires time, strength and patience.

* * *

This is the story of the ultimate cancer survivor, one who battled the disease for twenty-one years. A young Parsee lady with an eight-year-old son, whose family I knew well, developed breast cancer. Her Parsee husband, a doctor, immediately left her. She underwent surgery done by me (modified radical mastectomy) at the Parsee General Hospital, followed by appropriate oral chemotherapy. She was in remission for four years when she developed extensive lymph node metastasis. This was treated with prolonged chemotherapy by an oncologist, after which she was in remission for ten years. During these fourteen years, she would come faithfully and regularly to her follow-up appointments, often with her rapidly growing son. She was in total control of the prolonged disease, completely involved in her son's education and welfare, a busy stay-at-home, single mother, making the most of her life during her years of remission.

Around this time, fourteen years after the initial discovery of her breast cancer, she developed bone metastases. While she was being treated by the oncologist and radiologist, there was very marginal improvement, and after this poor response, she came to me for her follow-up appointment. She came alone this time to ask me, 'Doctor, is this the end of the road?' To keep hope alive, I said, 'I don't think so, you are a survivor.' Within a few weeks, well before her next scheduled follow-up, she came to see me again, this time for some advice. She had only vaguely heard, and not from any patient, of a lama in a monastery on the Indo-Tibet border, who could cure cancer. The entire family rubbished this news and forbade her from going so far based on unfounded information. She asked me if she should go. I mulled it over for a while. In my approach to medicine, I am holistic, and what cures, cures. For decades, I myself have used ghee and honey dressings for wounds, and pure carbolic acid as a healing agent. I do not accept that 'Western' medicine has all the answers. I also thought of the problems she might face travelling to the border of Tibet on her own, looking for an address on a piece of paper. After a long pause, I said, 'Dear, you simply *must* go.' She went and stayed there for a few months. On her return, the bone metastases were still there, not even partially regressed, but over time, had not progressed further. The important fact was that she was pain- and symptom-free—it was like her bone cancer had *never happened*. She remained in remission, a cancer survivor. During these long, repeated periods of remission, Khorshed and I drew close to the family. We were special guests at her son's wedding. Her son was twenty-eight at the time. A year later, she developed lung metastases and passed away, just a day after I visited her.

Closer to home, my cancer was dormant for two active, normal years, then multiple metastases appeared in both lungs. But one must be fair and pragmatic. My cancer was kind, almost benevolent. I have had over five years of a reasonably normal, productive life with an exceedingly aggressive form of the disease. Despite the prognosis, and my own surgical understanding of the inevitability that lies ahead, I have no reason to complain.

8

Surgery and Care of
the Elderly

If you pass by Warden Road in South Mumbai, you may notice a large and quite beautiful stone arch standing out in a sea of buildings. Drive under it and you will be led to the magnificent heritage structure that is the B.D. Petit Parsee General Hospital.

After the bubonic plague that ravaged Bombay at the start of the twentieth century, the Parsee community felt the need to establish a hospital exclusively for Parsees, which was unusual at the time as all Parsee charities thus far had been secular. In 1905, in response to Jehangir Bomanji Petit's appeal to the community for funds, his father Seth Bomanji Dinshawji Petit had offered his vast property, The Cumballa Hill Family Hotel, along with securities of 50,000 rupees for the hospital. A committee, formed after the appeal for funds to oversee the day-to-day running of the hospital, decided to name it after him. The Bombay Parsi Punchayet was tasked with the charge of the hospital and its grounds, merely as custodians, while all aspects of running the hospital fell within the ambit of an incorporated society registered in 1922. The foundation stone was laid in 1907 by the then Governor of Bombay, Sir George Clarke, and the hospital opened to the community in 1912.

Wards were divided into non-paying, part-paying and fully paying patients, although the ethos was to dispense equal and quality treatment to every patient, no matter their background. Social workers would assess the economic situation of the patient and admit them to the appropriate ward, so no family would need to pay more than they could afford. In addition to the Petit Family Trust, this truly patient-friendly charitable hospital was largely funded by contributions from the community, not only from India but from all over the world, including the Incorporated Zoroastrian Charity Funds of Hong Kong, Canton and Macau.

The hospital was active and running for fifty-five years when I was appointed Honorary Surgeon in 1967, but I was also working as a consultant paediatric surgeon at Wadia Children's Hospital, and as an assistant honorary surgeon at the JJ Hospital at the same time. Parsee General Hospital was my introduction to treating patients well into their seventies, eighties and even nineties. Initially, I would treat this elderly group the same way I treated all my patients, but the first thing my registrar, Dr Subhash Dalal taught me during my first resident post at the Wadia Children's Hospital was that 'you may treat an adult as a large child, but you can never treat a child as a small adult. The surgery of children is a science apart.' At Parsee General Hospital, I gradually became convinced, after stumbles, scares and failures, that surgery of the aged was also a science apart.

While the young could bounce back from a dangerous situation by virtue of their inherent vitality, the aged could slip into peril because of their innate vulnerability. I was trained to believe that every child must be treated like a child. But there was no one to guide, inform or instruct me to treat the aged as aged. Either this segment of the population was denied surgical care—deemed to be 'too old'—or were treated like others a few decades younger. This bias was evident even in the simplest of cases, like hernia. For example, older patients would not be advised elective hernia repairs, which resulted in emergency situations, and in turn, higher morbidity.

We also tended to assume that what all patients wanted at the end of their treatment was the same, but I slowly learnt, mainly by talking to them, that what the elderly desired the most was an improvement in their quality of life, a reinstatement of their independence, and a restoration of their dignity, among other things that younger people take for granted. For this age group, more lethal perhaps than the primary disease, are often the co-morbidities that affect several of their bodily functions. With increasing age, there is progressive deterioration in the performance of the heart, lungs, kidneys, metabolic system, fluid balance, temperature control, as also mental changes like cognition loss and dementia. Under normal conditions, unless the deterioration is severe, it is compatible with normal activity, but under conditions of stress imposed by illness, there could be a rapid exacerbation of the failure of one or more systems.

After years of treating geriatric patients at Parsee General Hospital, I believe that indications for surgery fall into four groups:

1. *To save life* such as in case of an intestinal obstruction or perforation or gangrene.
2. *To relieve symptoms* or pre-empt complications, as in recurrent episodes of acute cholecystitis, for example.
3. *To forestall complications*, as in the case of hernias.
4. *To improve the quality of life*, as with joint replacements.

But I often get the feeling that surgeons themselves are a major risk factor in the surgery of the aged. 65 per cent—or almost *two-thirds*—of post-operative deaths are *unrelated* to the surgery itself and are attributed to complications arising from co-morbidities, post-operative care and management.* Surgical treatment for the elderly has its own set of pitfalls, which pose a unique set of challenges for the surgeon to account for:

- *Their mental state*, which causes difficulties in diagnosis and management.

- *Low resilience and recuperative power*, which indicate both a limited capacity to withstand complications and slower recovery time.

- *A low margin of error*. The surgeon gets 'only one bite at the cherry,' and all treatment must be completed in the first attempt because the aged cannot withstand repeated intervention. A combination of patience and gentle handling will make older patients feel they are a part of the team, which helps them retain their cooperation and confidence, leading to better surgical outcomes.

- *Reaction to anaesthesia*, which should be regional (local) rather than general, where possible. This is because there is poor understanding of the demands of general anaesthesia from the aged. The old get hypothermic (cold) very rapidly in the cold OT. To assess respiratory function, pre-anaesthesia tests need to be done. When I started surgery on the aged, the standard practice was to ask the patient to blow out a lit match held six inches from their open mouth. Now, of course, there are far

---

* T.E. Udwadia, 1988, Surgery in the Aged, Pathological and Physiological Considerations, Annals of the National Academy of Medical Sciences 24: 203-215.

more sophisticated methods, but that was and remains a remarkably reliable test.

- *Altering approaches to pain management.* Analgesics are preferable over sedation, which depresses the cough reflex and coupled with reduced tolerance to the dose of sedation, could even result in permanent sleep! Management of pain in the elderly is a new specialty.

I cannot adequately stress the importance of teamwork between specialities in post-operative surgical care for the aged. Essentials for safe recovery include careful pre-operative preparation, healthy apprehension of and attention to co-morbidities, optimal surgery, keeping the surgeon's ego completely at bay, hawk-eyed post-operative care, rehabilitation and physiotherapy. The surgeon must also account for slower-than-usual healing when it comes to response to suture materials, for example.

Additionally, Intensive Care Units must be used as infrequently as possible; the old get frightened and disoriented in the ICU setting. If the case is indeed terminal, surgeons should know when to ease off treatment, and not prolong the misery of the patient. No sight could be sadder than a geriatric patient in the ICU with a tube in every opening of the body—in a vain effort to anchor them to earth. In our zeal to serve the aged, let us never forget that a vital part of our duty is to ensure that they have a dignified end.

The unexpected and exponential increase in this population is a common problem for all countries as it has put a strain on economies, and most of all, has created unique problems for the aged themselves, both medical and humanitarian. Globally, it is estimated that those over the age of sixty will exceed 1.4 billion in 2030 and 2.1 billion in 2050.[*] Of these 2 billion, 75 per cent will be in Low- or Middle-Income Countries (MLIC) like India. The percentage rise in the aged population of Indians over ten years from 2010–2020 was 38.4 per cent, whereas the rise in total population was 12.4 per cent.[†] Additionally, The Indian Council of Medical Research reports that the cancer burden in India, with the increasing percentage of aged, will jump to 29.8 million by 2025.[‡] The economic impact of this exponential rise is incalculable, considering that we cannot even address the problems of the present population. The situation is far worse in rural areas. And statistics do not adequately portray the travails of the individual sufferer.

The younger the surgeon or doctor, the more important it is for them to get actively involved in geriatric care because as they grow into their practice, the number of aged will increase exponentially, and they will need to cope with this population out of necessity. Better medical education, increased social and financial support, more training and commitment in the care of the aged is the need of the hour.

Over the past fifty years at the Parsee General Hospital, I have perhaps spent as much time talking to the elderly as

---

[*] 'Ageing', WHO. Available at: https://www.who.int/health-topics/ageing#tab=tab_1.

[†] S. Irudaya Rajan, *Ageing in India* (Mumbai: Centre for Enquiry into Health and Allied Themes (CEHAT), 2006). Available at: https://www.cehat.org/cehat/uploads/files/ageing(1).pdf.

[‡] Priyanka Sharma, 'India's cancer burden to rise to 29.8 million in 2025: ICMR report', LiveMint, 13 May 2022. Available at: https://www.livemint.com/science/health/indias-cancer-burden-to-rise-to-29-8-million-in-2025-icmr-report-11652382169284.html.

treating them, and I find their needs to be reasonable and meagre. All they want is:

- *A good quality of life.* Chronic diseases, co-morbidities, financial constraints, changes in family dynamics, customs and mental stress—all threaten their quality of life. They wish to continue the limited joys they have, have their drink (not allowed by doctors), shuffle over to a food stall, or in the case of Parsees, read the *Jam-e-Jamshed* and abuse the Hospital's Trustees.
- *Reduction or stoppage in the progression of their conditions, both physical and mental.* This could be done by educating them about the concept of prevention, which includes imparting information about good nutrition, management of their co-morbidities, daily and simple exercises like walking, and basic physiotherapy to maintain optimal use of their lungs and muscles. In the aged, the margin of safety is so narrow that prevention is far easier than cure.
- *Social interaction.* Advancing age brings with it the increasing loss of children's support, the loss of a life partner, health issues, depression, decreased income, loss of mobility, social isolation, loneliness, loss of vision and hearing, all of which could lead to further deterioration of mental and physical health. For example, loneliness carries in its wake a string of conditions like anxiety and depression, and increases the risk of dementia and other co-morbidities. It also causes emotional pain, which activates the same stress responses as physical

pain. Mobility is essential to maintaining some degree of social contact, and prophylactic exercises, walkers and other means can go a long way in helping with that.

Over the decades, I have realized how limited the appreciation was among surgeons and anaesthetists of the fact that taking care of the aged was a different beast that needed special understanding. This lack of understanding is not unique to India but rather, is a worldwide tragedy for 'there is an enormous need for competence in the care of the geriatric surgical patients in the majority of hospitals worldwide' and a 'need for dramatically increasing geriatric competence among surgeons and anaesthetists'.[*]

A part of the problem of the aged is our lack of acceptance, even today, of the fact that geriatrics—the science of the overall care of the aged—needs as much recognition in teaching hospitals and universities as any other specialty. While some hospitals like the JJ Hospital are planning postgraduate courses in geriatric medicine, education in geriatrics is still largely overlooked, not only in India but in most countries. The surgeon who acquires some experience, and perhaps wisdom, in the care of the elderly patient, will become a more versatile clinician, a more humane doctor, and perhaps a more tranquil recipient of the inevitable truth that he or she is also ageing. I speak from first-hand experience. At the age of eighty-eight, I realize how quickly time has flown.

---

[*] Gabriella Bitelli, 'Preoperative Evaluation of the Elderly Surgical Patient and an Anaesthesia Challenges in the XXIst century', *Ageing Clinical and Experimental Research*, 2018 (published online 14 February 2018).

Developments in geriatric care and medicine will require government planning but the individual clinician can do a lot too. Growing old is a natural and inevitable part of life, yet all old people are not about to die! Across millennia, the aged have been sought for their wisdom and counsel, as we learn from the ancient writings of the Greeks, the Romans and the Vedas. They are a rich gateway to the past and have lived experiences that cannot be replicated. If you have older people in your life or as your patients, ask them questions, seek their advice, listen to their stories, and learn what you can from them. What they have to say could make you wiser.

9

Some Joy, Some Pride, Some Stupidity

When I was young, I was like most boys, collecting things for the sheer joy of collecting them. Some of my friends would collect cigarette packets, others Coca-Cola bottle caps. The clever ones would collect stamps, but as for me, I collected marbles. I only had ten, but each one was special—vivid colours trapped in glass and frozen in time. My most valuable marble was a 'bunto', three times the size of the others. These objects may not have been valuable or relevant to anyone else, but they were precious to me.

In my very average academic career, I collected precisely two awards. The first was for topping English in the 1949 SSC exam, and the second was the Dr Shirvalkar Medal for Clinical Medicine, as an undergraduate at GS Medical College in 1954. Much to my disappointment, I didn't get the surgery medal, and I felt that the only reason I had won the medal in medicine was because the external examiner was my father's friend.

But over the course of a surgical career that spanned seven decades, I have collected more things along the way that have been of special value to me. Some of these have made me proud, some have brought me immense joy, and some have been lessons that have humbled me. I fully acknowledge all the numerous errors I made when I was trying something new or different—I'm not ashamed of them, they were a crucial part of my surgical career growth. What dismays me is my own stupidity, my not doing what was necessary because of laziness or the inability to visualize the potential importance of what I was exposed to. 'Some Joy, Some Pride, Some Stupidity' is a chequered collection of unexpected and unasked for honours, nuggets of wisdom, and some mistakes made along the way.

The Hunterian Lecturer, 1984

I was failed in the MS exam of 1960 by the examiner Professor S.S. Anand, who added salt to my wounds by saying that I should feel proud to have been failed by a Hunterian lecturer—whatever that meant. At the time, I did not know or care about what a Hunterian lecturer was; all I could think about was that I had failed my wife and newborn child. While the desire to pull out the examiner's beard strand by strand faded over time, what he had said struck a chord within me. In the days before the internet, the only way to keep abreast of developments in my field was to read surgical journals. One night, I was reading the *Journal of the Royal College of Surgeons of England*, when I spotted a notice for the election to the office of the 1984 Hunterian Lecturer. Applicants had to submit original, clinically related and unpublished work. The last date for receiving applications at the college office was only ten days away.

Although my daughter Dinaz, my 'home secretary', was fast asleep, I gently woke her up and asked her to type an initial draft of the application that I dictated. She did it as best as she could, leaving out words she did not understand. I worked on the application for the next three days, redrafting and making corrections until I was satisfied. Next came the problem of getting a good printout. My college friend, Chondi Gupta, the Medical Director of Burroughs Wellcome (India), said he could have his office do it, but it was the weekend. On Monday morning, Dinaz skipped her classes at law college and took the draft to Chondi, who sent me the printout. After minor corrections, the application was ready, but the deadline was two days away. How was I to get it to England in time?

Air India came to the rescue. As senior surgeon to the airline, I was in touch with several of their staff. Colleen Bhiladwala, the chief airhostess of the airline, and her fiancé Zafar Hai, were my patients, and later my friends. Colleen's response was immediate—she would give the application to the senior airhostess on that night's flight to London. It would be in the Royal College of Surgeons' office on the next day. And I didn't even have to pay for postage stamps!

A few months later, I got a reply from the college council, informing me I had been elected the Hunterian Lecturer and that the date for my lecture was 22 March 1984. The date suited Khorshed and me perfectly. Dinaz was getting married, and she and Khorshed were planning a shopping trip to London. We rented an apartment and while the two of them shopped, I worked on my lecture. One day, alone in the apartment, I had a panic attack, and for good reason. I, an unknown Indian surgeon, still in my forties, had to give a lecture to the cream of English surgeons in the Mecca of English surgery, The Royal College of Surgeons of England. Moreover, the title of my lecture was 'Peritoneoscopy (Laparoscopy) for Surgeons'. In those days, laparoscopy was anathema to all surgeons, and the only two people who I knew practised it, were my mentor, George Berci—the father of all endoscopy—in Los Angeles, and Alfred Cuchieri from Dundee, who still continues to break new ground.

No one can beat the British at pomp and pageantry. Before the lecture, I was taken to a large room where I was made to wear a special college gown. Members of the council and senior fellows were also similarly gowned. The chairman for my Hunterian Lecture was the Vice President of the College, Professor Harold Ellis, soon to be knighted by the Queen. The procession to the main hall began with Professor Ellis and I at the head and all the gowned surgeons walking behind us in pairs. Dinaz ran forward to take my picture as we walked past the statue of John Hunter, after whom the lecture had been instituted in 1810. The butterflies in my stomach grew to the size of sparrows as I entered the hall and was introduced to the audience. Embarrassed by Professor Ellis's fulsome praise, I looked down at the floor. When I finally looked up, I burst into a huge smile from ear to ear, for I could see several brown faces, scattered all over the hall in the sea of white, many of whom I recognized.

These faces belonged to former students of JJ Hospital, who had gathered from all over England, Scotland, Wales, and Ireland to ensure that I felt welcome and at home. Rajiv

Chinoy, my former resident surgeon at the JJ, had individually contacted (as there was no WhatsApp in those days) most JJ residents in the UK. Many were pathologists, ophthalmologists and psychiatrists, some of whom had not even seen me until then. *Such is the unique spirit of JJ.* I acknowledged them all with a quick wave of my hand, thanked JJ and started my lecture. By now, I was euphoric, and my lecture went like a dream, and was published in the college journal.* After the college formalities at the end of the lecture, we 'brownies' crossed the road to go over to the pub. It was so crowded that many from our group had to stand outside on the pavement as we all raised our glasses to toast Grant Medical College and JJ Hospital.

Emeritus Professor of Surgery at JJ Hospital, 1994

While I retired in 1992 as Professor of Surgery at Grant Medical College and JJ Hospital, I was given an extension to ensure that JJ would not lose the MS seats with me. (Every professor has MS students under them. As the senior-most, I had the most. If I left too early, those students would be derecognized and by staying on for over a year, they could then be redistributed to continue their studies under other professors). I left over a year later and was soon appointed by a government gazette order as the Emeritus Professor of Surgery at Grant Medical College and JJ Hospital, the first Emeritus Professor of Surgery in its more-than-100-

---

* T.E. Udwadia, 'Peritoneoscopy for Surgeons', *Annals of the Royal College of Surgeons of England*, 68, 1986, pp. 125–129.

year-old history. I have often wondered why they gave me
this honour, but then thought it could have been the result
of the international recognition the hospital received with
the introduction of laparoscopy in 1972, as well as the first
laparoscopic cholecystectomy in the developing world in
1990, both of which were conducted at the JJ Hospital.

Society of American Gastrointestinal Endoscopic Surgeons (SAGES) Millennium Award for Surgical Innovations, 2000

In 1999, I received a letter from the honours committee of
SAGES informing me that I had been awarded the SAGES
Millennium Award 2000 for Surgical Innovation. I was elated!
Part of the honour was to give an eponymous lecture and I
decided to fly high with the preposterous title, 'One World,
One People, One Surgery'. My lecture was months away, so
I thought I had plenty of time to prepare. But work and travel
gobbled up time, and suddenly, I was just left with a month
to go. Then something happened that had never happened
before. I developed a severe case of writer's block. I could not
produce a single usable word! As one month shrank to two
weeks, I began to panic. Around this time, one of Mumbai's
most famous theatre personalities, 'adman' Alyque Padamsee
came to me for a post-operative check-up. When I told him
about my problem, he asked me to meet him for lunch two
days later at the Royal Bombay Yacht Club.

For two hours, Alyque interrogated me like a lawyer cross-
examining a difficult witness. He wanted to know about my

passions, my views and the message I wanted to convey. After the grilling, I was exhausted, but he was still bubbly. He told me to go home and recall every bit of our two-hour conversation. 'You'll then have your lecture,' he promised. Indeed, the lecture was ready in three days. When I phoned to thank Alyque, he said that he had done nothing, and that I already had the lecture in me. The lecture was well-received and was printed in *Surgical Endoscopy*, the SAGES journal.[*]

Honorary Fellowship of the Association of Rural Surgeons of India, 2004

I am a city surgeon, but in my mission to spread awareness about the benefits of diagnostic laparoscopy and later, laparoscopic surgery, I travelled from 1975 to small towns, rural areas and even tribal regions. I learnt far more than I taught in my travels into the interiors, and invariably returned home humbled by the strength of our rural surgeons. The Association of Rural Surgeons of India, in recognition for my support for rural surgery, made me an Honorary Fellow of the Association of Rural Surgeons at their Annual Conference at Vapi, Gujarat in 2004. I regard this fellowship as one of my most prized honours. I felt humbled and honoured at being accepted as one of them, for I have always considered rural surgeons to be the backbone of Indian surgery.

---

[*] T.E. Udwadia, 'One World, One People, One Surgery', *Surgical Endoscopy*, 15, 2001, pp. 337–43.

Honorary Member of the German Society of Visceral (Abdominal) Surgery, 2006

This Society not only requested me to give a keynote lecture on the futuristic topic, 'Navigating Laparoscopic Surgery Over the Next Ten Years', at their Annual Congress in Berlin, but they also gave me a monetary award. The icing on the cake, to my surprise, was being made an honorary member of the prestigious German Society of Visceral Surgery at the inaugural ceremony. My lecture was published in the *Langenbeck's Archives of Surgery*, the world's oldest surgical journal.*

Honorary Fellowship of The American College of Surgeons (ACS), 2010

The ACS is the world's largest surgical body, comprising surgeons from Canada and the United States. Every year, its honours committee selects a few surgeons worldwide working outside North America, who have made significant contributions to the field of surgery, to be their honorary fellows. The presentation is held at the packed opening function, with near-British levels of pomp and pageantry, complete with gowns, processions, et al. The citations of the honorary fellows are read on stage (mine was read by Professor John Hunter), thereafter, the collar is placed on the awardees' gowns, the president says a few words of congratulations, and then finally, the award is presented on stage. It's quite a dramatic ceremony

---

* T.E. Udwadia, 'Navigating Laparoscopic Surgery into the Next Decade', *Langenbeck's Archives of Surgery*, 392, 2007, pp. 99–104.

and honorary fellows are granted a permanent place in the pantheon of the ACS.

SAGES George Berci Lifetime Achievement Award, 2013

Considered to be the ultimate award in laparoscopy, this is the highest honour that can be bestowed by SAGES and is named after my mentor, George Berci, the father of all endoscopy. This is not an annual award but given only as and when a recipient is found worthy. As I got off the stage after my acceptance speech, George Berci came up to me and gave me a warm hug. We were both moist-eyed. As I said in my acceptance speech, while brandishing the award, 'Ladies and gentlemen, with due respect to the American College of Surgeons and Her Majesty Queen Elizabeth II, this award surely takes the cake.'

* * *

But it wasn't always smooth sailing. The second part of this chapter is devoted to my many considerable stupidities; stupidities that make me shudder every time I remember them.

Research at JJ Hospital—A Missed Opportunity

In 1963, after being trained under a research-oriented chief—Professor Sen at KEM—I joined as Assistant Professor in the Department of Surgery at the JJ Hospital. I quickly observed that there was not only a complete absence of research activity at the JJ Hospital, but also antipathy towards it.

I wanted to continue my discipline of conducting research and decided to focus my efforts on one of the most common and most painful of anal diseases, Fissure-in-Ano. The external anal sphincter muscle is shaped like a tennis racket with the handle pointing to the back end of the anus and, as this area is not supported by the sphincter (muscle), it is prone to tearing during the passage of a hard stool, leading to a fissure. This, I felt, was the result of faulty evolution—homo sapiens became erect without adequately adapting to the new posture, causing problems like hernia and varicose veins. I spent two years working on the research project titled 'The Prophylaxis (Prevention) of Fissure-in-Ano',[*] which documented and validated a simple procedure to prevent it.

The idea of doing the study first came to me when I was preparing a lecture on the anatomy of the anal canal. I recalled conversations that Khorshed and I had had, where she used to tell me how constipated she and all her friends were at Presentation Convent, her school in Kodaikanal, yet how free they were of any problems because they were taught to exert upward pressure in the rear midline on the skin behind the anus with one finger when passing a hard stool. I paid no attention to what she said, thinking it was an old wives' tale. But what if it wasn't? What if something that simple could prevent a very common disease that becomes chronic and painful in later life?

---

[*] T.E. Udwadia, 'The Prophylaxis of Fissure-in-Ano', *Indian Journal of Surgery* (1978, 40, (11): 560).

I decided to investigate this further—a process that took two years. The research on this procedure was multidimensional, completely original and was, to date, the best research I have ever done in any hospital. In the first arm of my study, the anatomy department of Grant Medical College helped me study anal anatomy and function thoroughly. I had the good fortune to get Piroja Irani (later the wife of Dr Noshir Wadia) to willingly support me with several Electromyography (EMG) Stimulation studies on the various muscles of the anal canal at rest, while active, and most importantly, during the simulated passage of a hard stool, the second arm of the study. For the third and most important arm, I roped in friendly and willing interns who had been my unit's students during their surgical posting, for clinical trials. Severe constipation was induced in them using medication and then observing the efficacy of finger pressure at the posterior midline to prevent the occurrence of Fissure-in-Ano. The clinical trial supplemented the findings of the anatomy and EMG studies, and fully confirmed the efficacy of this procedure.

After two years of this study, I submitted my work for a prize for surgeons below the age of forty-five. I did not win. But not winning the prize was not why I consider this as evidence of my stupidity. Rather, because I was childish, immature or annoyed at not having won, I failed to pursue the research any further. Even though I had validation that this method worked, I let an award determine its significance. Foolishly, I just stopped working on it! I withdrew from the opportunity of popularizing a simple procedure that could greatly alleviate the suffering of affected individuals. I mention this study in these pages with the hope that perhaps someone else could pick up the study from where it left off, and possibly provide relief to millions from what could be an easily preventable condition.

Laparoscopy, 1980—The Blinkered, Stupid Surgeon

In 1980, I took a sabbatical to spend time observing the laparoscopic gynaecologist Kurt Semm. I was in the OT for every procedure he did. At the time, everyone who did laparoscopy held the telescope with their left hand. But across more than seventy cases, Semm used a gadget he had created that was attached to the operation table, kept the telescope in a fixed position, and freed his left hand. While I observed how masterful his technique was, I could not pinpoint what was making the difference. I would discuss his procedures, view his collection of thousands of colour slides, but somewhere I was not seeing the big picture. I only belatedly realized what the game-changer was—by keeping the telescope fixed, he could use *both* hands for laparoscopy. How could I have missed that?!

Had I the common sense to study his gadget and understand how it was made, I would have learnt how to use both my hands for laparoscopy, and could have, over time, perhaps performed the *world's* first laparoscopic cholecystectomy! Semm, a gynaecologist, performed the world's first laparoscopic appendectomy that same year. His German association forbade him to do such heterodox surgery in the future and his paper was rejected until 1983 when it was published in an American journal. It did not make me feel less stupid to know that scores of gynaecologists who followed me on sabbaticals with Semm

(I was the only surgeon), too failed to see the potential of his telescope holder!

The Changing Face of Abdominal Tuberculosis and Giant Hernias—Unpublished Studies

I carried out a mammoth clinical study at JJ Hospital on abdominal tuberculosis, wherein I studied and compared all cases of the disease across three discrete decades (from 1963 to 1972, from 1973 to 1982, and from 1983 to 1992) to understand how it evolved, thereby documenting its changing face. There was nothing original or clever about what I did, but the study was a good statistical and clinical review. However, while I presented this work at both national and international conferences, I failed to publish it. It remains a regret because it would have made a good reference paper on a common disease in India.

I feel the same way about not publishing work I had done on giant hernias. Today's herniologists may perhaps not be able to imagine the number, size and variety of the giant hernias surgeons saw in the 1950s, 60s, 70s, 80s or even 90s, that were left untreated. Some had more than 30 per cent of the abdominal contents in the hernia. Replacing the hernia contents would endanger respiration—intra-abdominal pressure would increase after replacing the hernial contents into the abdomen, severely compromising both the respiratory and cardiovascular systems.

I realized that to minimize morbidity or mortality, two essential steps needed to be taken:

1. Adapt the abdominal cavity to receive the hernial contents by distending it, by instilling air into the cavity and maintaining it at a pressure of 12 mmHg for a few weeks. Since I was doing this routinely for laparoscopy, this was not a problem.
2. At time of closure of the abdomen, minimize the tension of closure (to minimize intra-abdominal pressure) by making release incisions in muscles and fascia, like a tailor opening the sides to make the garment looser. The release incisions I made were not as complex and extensive as those used by herniologists today, but they were the earliest efforts to minimize intra-abdominal pressure.

This work was presented at national and international conferences with operative slides and videos, but sadly was not published. Doing so could have helped map the historical progression of the treatment of giant hernias from the past to the present, with its more complex approach.

Having said that, I do not like to sound as if I am making excuses, but publishing a paper in the pre-internet era was a difficult and tedious task. The only way to get a reference was to go to the library, take out the huge, dusty annual volume of *Index Medicus*, and pore over the small print till you found it. To obtain just three references could, on a bad day, take longer than completing an operation list. Surgeons publishing papers today by the truckload may not appreciate what an easy wicket they are on.

Each one of my unpardonable stupidities mentioned here (and I have included but a few) are, for me, horrific. Yet, the worst way of treating blunders is to brush them under the carpet. They deserve to be aired and highlighted in public as a clear reminder that stupidity should not become a habit.

But with childish vanity, let me talk of the joys of my long journey. Small things please small minds, and I gush over the awards mentioned in these pages, like I did over my marbles as a child, though they are not, to most, a big deal. The honours cited here (and some not mentioned like the Honorary Member of the Society of Endoscopic and Laparoscopic Surgeons of Asia [ELSA], or induction into the Hall of Fame, Asia Pacific Hernia Society [APHS]), are those that would not be considered big news, but they mattered to me because they were given by bodies I respect and admire for their impeccable scientific quality. They were unexpected and unasked for, bestowed by organizations that make decisions that could not be influenced.

Epilogue

The epilogue was 'written' in two parts, at two different times, in two very different circumstances, as will become apparent to the reader.

The first part was written around mid-November 2022, when Dr Udwadia was in relatively good health. He was going to Breach Candy Hospital to see his patients, playing golf from time to time, visiting IMMAST occasionally, and phoning his friends to chat. There was a spring in his step and the usual twinkle in his eyes. His voice was upbeat, there was optimism in the air and the hope that he would get some more months of near-normal life.

The second part was dictated over several days to his daughter Dinaz between the end of December 2022 and early January 2023, from his bed in Breach Candy Hospital. His health had deteriorated significantly by mid-December. His beloved wife Khorshed broke her hip on 24 December and was in Breach Candy Hospital and he wanted to be near her, so he too moved there. He knew by now that the end was nigh. He was supported by non-invasive ventilation and drugged with fentanyl. His words barely a whisper, occasionally incoherent, were interpreted as best she could by Dinaz, and those are the words that you will read in the second part of the epilogue.

One Way to Live, I realize, turned out to be a brief sketch of my life and thoughts, but in no way implies or suggests that this is for anyone else a way to live. When I think back, I realize how very unique and singular each individual life is, and each to his or her own way of living. That said, every life merges into one universal pool of all humanity—birth, life and the onward journey. As a child at school, I collected marbles, but those who collected cigarette packets had one more valuable packet than all the rest. It was a violet-coloured one with a man in a tailcoat and top hat. The name of the cigarette was 'Passing Show'. I feel that this cigarette packet told the story of life. We strut about in our finery on the stage of life for a few brief moments in time, then move on to give our place to the next wave, a passing show that merges into eternity, impressing the impermanence of all we do and desire, and the futility of taking life too seriously in the endless cycle of time.

My family has been the reason I have emerged well from surgery. The children have dropped everything and flown in from different corners of the world to be with me through difficult times. I feel bad about the problems I am creating for

149

them, and I hope they know how much it means to Khorshed and me to have them around, flying in during these difficult times, disrupting their family, professional and personal lives.

But without Khorshed, there would be no me. Through all these decades, she has been my rock; steadfast, solid, soft, loving. She would see me off every morning after a rushed breakfast, stand at the window to wave me good luck and stay there to say a prayer as I left. From a flighty girl who would take off her high heels and run after a Victoria carriage when we were courting, she evolved into a happy wife, mother and housewife. She had her little tricks to make sure that laughter was a prime feature of our household. She would thump a Turkish March on the piano, or glide into a gentle Chopin, sometimes keeping the neighbours awake and tapping their toes. She made special dishes once or twice a week, nervously waiting for the verdict on her cooking. She was a complete homebody—she went for only one ladies' coffee party, but came home and said it was scary because all they did, she said, was say nasty things about everyone who was not at the party. She enjoyed wearing new clothes, going out with me late in the evenings to friends' homes or more often, just the two of us would go to Bombelli's, The Society at The Ambassador, or for pani-puri at Chowpatty. In addition to being a fulltime housewife, she was a fulltime florist for fifty-five years, running her two landmark flower shops by the name of 'Pushpa Milan', one of the earliest and longest-serving members of Interflora.

Khorshed's loss of hearing has gradually increased. As time has gone by, she has become much quieter, no longer the life of the party. Often seen by most as a minor disability, this condition does not evoke the same level of empathy as one would have for someone with loss of vision or a limb. I get every new hearing aid for her with the hope, if not the expectation, that it would help her. From an extroverted, bubbly girl who, till her early eighties, could rock with her friends by bursting into her own version of 'There's a rich Maharajah of Magador . . . who had rubies and pearls, and the loveliest girls . . .' she has slowly become quieter, introverted and, to my dismay, unwilling to socialize. Wherever she goes, she is engulfed by silence. She comes out only to make me happy. Her great joy and pleasure, music, is denied to her. She seldom plays the piano, and only does so after repeated requests and persuasion. Only someone who has experienced their loved one go through hearing loss will know what it really means. The happy hours of conversation we shared have now reduced to a few words, pats and hugs. When we drive home from social gatherings, she asks me, 'What were all those people saying?' I have a standard reply to which she gives a smile and a nod: 'They said nothing of any consequence'.

With time to contemplate over the years, I do feel a well-lived life is good preparation for our inevitable exit. A life where the pursuit of joy, the permanence of friendship, the acceptance of any success as a gift from above and counting one's blessings, are far more enriching than counting one's acquisitions. Having been clearly informed by my doctors that they have no further treatment options for my cancer, I strive to make each day count. I spend as much quality time as I can with Khorshed, continue my OPD clinic at Breach Candy

Hospital, take joy that my golf skills are improving, keep the hope of travel alive, live my life, face my cancer. Brave words. But I do hope I do not buckle under in the last slog overs at the end of the innings. My dream is to hit a sixer off the last ball. Can I?

* * *

The deterioration of my condition has progressed rapidly. Early morning on Christmas Eve, Khorshed fell and fractured her hip. With Khorshed in the hospital, common sense dictated I be admitted as well, for I needed to be near her. The morphine administered to me made me feel terrible—drowsy, confused and incapable of coherent thought. I was put on a BIPAP breathing machine with constant high-flow oxygen. All I did was sleep with incapacitating constipation and increasing disorientation. On explaining my predicament, the doctors told me they would increase the dose of morphine, which made me feel worse, and hastened my deterioration. I would have preferred to die.

But miracles never stop falling from above. Two young doctors, Shamali Poojari and Sumith Surendran, from the palliative care team at Tata Memorial Hospital, collaborated with Rushad, and advised substituting morphine with fentanyl. Considering the state I was in, any change was welcome. I now feel appreciatively better—more alert, aware of my surroundings, and able to think. I feel I have a new lease on life and have become brighter, cheerful, interested in my surroundings and activities, ready to live again.

Of course, I know the reality of the situation, but I am grateful to grab the remainder of time on my terms. Khorshed was operated upon on 29 December and has fortunately recovered. God in His bountiful mercy, created the best evening of our lives. Khorshed came to my room and we had dinner together. It was the most beautiful dinner we have ever had. I hope we have a few more days like this together, reminiscing about our life, which was truly made in Heaven, and where for sixty-four years, we have lived together as one person in our joys, in our problems, in our enthusiasm, in all that has made our life a life of a lifetime.

We could not have asked for more. We could not have received more. We could not have appreciated our time together more. And we could not have praised the Lord more. I look forward to a few more evenings of togetherness and time to reminisce. Love has no beginning and no end.

Dr Udwadia passed away on 7 January 2023, surrounded by his children.

Acknowledgements

I would like to thank Khorshed, my partner of over sixty years and by far my better half, as well as my children Rushad, Dinaz and Ashad, who have always loved and supported me without question, along with my entire family, including my grandchildren-in-law, who are my joy. To my brother Darius, who, while being sceptical about my book projects, nevertheless always remained completely supportive, thank you. I would also like to use this opportunity to express my gratitude to my mother and father, who taught me, as St Paul wrote, to 'Build your house on rock, not sand.' The foundation is everything.

I am deeply indebted to Titoo Ahluwalia, my friend of over forty years. Supportive, critical and honest, he has been the quiet force behind this book. Early in life, I learnt that friends are forever. Over the years, Titoo showed me how. I would also like to acknowledge the efforts of Gayatri Pahlajani, who is in her second innings as my editor for this book. She is erudite and provides sharp, relevant inputs. I strongly recommend her to all struggling authors.

I wish Dorab Sopariwala—my friend for the last few years, who has helped me with both books—had come into my life earlier. Master of the English language, he has brought precision to the book. He is a true-blue Parsee, what more can I say? I would also like to express my appreciation to Deepraj Bhandarkar, my colleague of over three decades, who provided reference material, additional readings and statistics at short notice, promptly and happily.

This book would not have been possible without the only two people who can read my handwriting—Sanika Sawant, who typed out the entire first book, and Megha Patil, my secretary for over ten years at ceMAST. Both have worked overtime on this book, and I am grateful to them for their patience and precision.

And finally, to the team at Penguin Random House India, and especially Ankit Juneja, thank you for your understanding, patience and compassion throughout this project.

All good things come from above.